Poultry Welfare Issues

Beak Trimming

Poultry Welfare Issues

Beak Trimming

Edited by P.C. Glatz

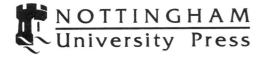

NOTTINGHAM
University Press

Nottingham University Press
Manor Farm, Main Street, Thrumpton
Nottingham NG11 0AX, United Kingdom
www.nup.com

NOTTINGHAM

First published 2005
© The contributors named in the list of contributors

British Library Cataloguing in Publication Data
Poultry Welfare Issues - Beak Trimming
I Glatz, P.C.

ISBN   1-904761-20-8

Disclaimer

Every reasonable effort has been made to ensure that the material in this book is true, correct, complete and appropriate at the time of writing. Nevertheless, the publishers and authors do not accept responsibility for any omission or error, or for any injury, damage, loss or financial consequences arising from the use of the book.

Typeset by Nottingham University Press, Nottingham
Printed and bound by Hobbs the Printers, Hampshire, England

Preface

Since the release of the Brambell Committee report on welfare in the UK in 1965 discussion on the welfare of beak-trimmed birds has continued unabated. The Brambell Committee recommended that beak-trimming should be stopped immediately in caged birds and within two years for non-caged birds. Nearly four decades later and beak-trimming is still a common practice in the poultry industry, despite years of research examining solutions to avoid its use.

There is a wealth of scientific information on the welfare of beak-trimmed birds, beak-trimming methods and alternatives to beak-trimming. The purpose of this volume is to consolidate this information.

The book commences with a chapter which outlines the methods of beak-trimming and how the practice is used to avoid injuries and deaths caused by cannibalism, bullying and feather and vent pecking. Most of the beak-trimming practised involves the partial removal of the upper and lower beak using an electrically heated blade that cuts and cauterises the beak and blunts the beak enough so that pecking cannot do any great damage. New methods have been developed using infrared and laser technology, which require further development and evaluation.

The ethical questions that need to be asked about beak-trimming are explored in the second chapter and discuss whether beak-trimming is fair and whether it is necessary. The poultry industry argues that beak-trimming is fair, because the consequences to the birds of cannibalism in untrimmed flocks are unpleasant. The counter arguments against beak-trimming are based on the premise that modern farming should not need to resort to mutilations in order to correct for over-intensification.

The major welfare concern associated with beak-trimming is that partial removal of the beak may cause acute and chronic pain due to tissue damage and nerve injury resulting in changes to bird behaviour. These aspects are examined in three chapters; the first is devoted to examining the major phases in the pain response associated with beak-trimming; the second details the complex changes in beak anatomy that occur after beak-trimming and the third discusses the changes in the physiology and behaviour of birds after beak-trimming. These chapters are followed by an assessment of the production advantages and disadvantages of beak-trimming for the industry. Factors such as liveability, plumage quality, feed efficiency and economics are compared in untrimmed and beak-trimmed birds.

Physical damage to the birds, suffocation through incorrect penning and handling procedures, acute blood loss due to bleeding, checks in bird growth and loss of flock uniformity are issues discussed in a chapter examining handling and health issues associated with beak-trimming.

The final chapter is devoted to examining the alternative strategies, which have been researched to avoid the need for beak-trimming. One potential method to eradicate the desire of birds to feather peck is to fit string enrichment devices in cages to promote natural behaviours and reduce boredom. This aspect is discussed in a section on environmental enrichment. String enrichment devices are now being used routinely on a number of farms in Europe.

Interest in the genetics of feather pecking and cannibalism has grown in the last few decades and a genetic solution might be more sustainable and cost effective than beak-trimming and environmental modifications. A section in the last chapter is devoted to discussing the genetic differences in the rate of feather pecking, quality of plumage and mortality from cannibalism between populations of domestic fowl. There is accumulating evidence supporting the existence of additive genetic effects underlying feather pecking behaviour. Recent discovery of quantative trait loci for performing and receiving feather pecking may offer the opportunity for enhancing the selection intensity.

Dietary solutions are discussed in a section examining the role of insoluble fibre in the diet to reduce the mortality from cannibalism. To reduce the occurrence of cannibalism, the authors in this section suggest that laying hens should be fed diets containing high-insoluble fibre such as millrun, oat hulls, rice hulls and lucerne meal.

Another section in the last chapter discusses light intensity, colour and quality in sheds and its impact on aggressive pecking and stereotype behaviours in hens. Low light intensity during the chick rearing stage discourages development of pecking vices. As light intensity increases there is a greater risk of cannibalism.

An aspect discussed in the last chapter suggests that correct management of body weight and minimising flock weight distributions can have a profound influence on the incidence of mucosal tearing, cloacal haemorrhage and subsequent cannibalism in multiple bird cages.

A potential solution to replace the need for beak-trimming is to apply an abrasive strip in the feed trough to blunt the tips of the beaks of laying hens. This has resulted in lower mortality caused by pecking behaviour.

The final section in the last chapter discusses the role of anti pecking devices and stock wound sprays to reduce subsequent cannibalism in hens. Practical experience has shown that treating the everted vent of hens suffering vent trauma with a stock wound spray can prevent further pecking and rehabilitate hens.

This volume will be of interest to welfare groups, policy makers, scientists, industry leaders and students of poultry science who wish to acquaint themselves with the welfare issues associated with beak-trimming and the potential solutions for reducing the need to beak-trim poultry.

Philip C. Glatz
Pig and Poultry Production Institute
Roseworthy, South Australia
January 2005

Contributors

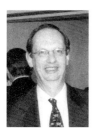

John L. Barnett
Animal Welfare Science Centre
Department of Primary Industries
600 Sneydes Road
Werribee 3030
Victoria
Australia

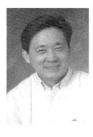

Heng-wei Cheng
125 S Russell Street
Poultry Science Building
Purdue University
West Lafayette
Indiana
USA 47907

Mingan Choct
School of Rural Science and Agriculture
University of New England
Armidale
New South Wales 2351
Australia

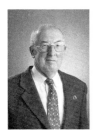

Arnold Elson
ADAS Gleadthorpe Poultry Research Centre
Meden Vale
Mansffield
Nottingham NG20 9PF
United Kingdom

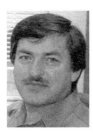

Philip C. Glatz
South Australian Research and Development Institute
Roseworthy Campus
University of Adelaide
Roseworthy
South Australia 5371
Australia

Contributors

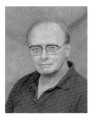

Neville G. Gregory
Silsoe Research Institute
Wrest Park
Silsoe
Bedfordshire MK454HS
United Kingdom

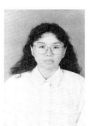

Sri Hartini
School of Rural Science and Agriculture
University of New England
Armidale
New South Wales 2351
Australia

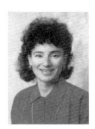

Patricia Y. Hester
125 S Russell Street
Poultry Science Building
Purdue University
West Lafayette
Indiana 47907
USA

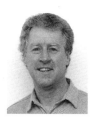

R. Bryan Jones
Welfare Biology Group
Roslin Institute
Roslin
Midlothian EH25 9PS
Scotland
UK

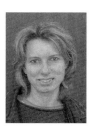

Ellen C. Jongman
Animal Welfare Science Centre
Department of Primary Industries
600 Sneydes Road
Werribee 3030
Victoria
Australia

Joergen B. Kjaer
Department of Animal Health and Welfare
Danish Institute of Agricultural Sciences
Research Centre Foulum
P.O. Box 50
DK-8830 Tjele
Denmark

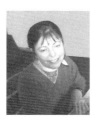

Christine A. Lunam
Department of Anatomy and Histology
and Centre for Neuroscience
Finders University
GPO Box 2100
Adelaide
SA 5001
Australia

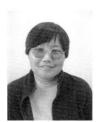

Zhihong H. Miao
South Australian Research and Development Institute
Roseworthy Campus
University of Adelaide
Roseworthy
South Australia 5371
Australia

Thea G.C.M. Fiks-van Niekerk
Applied Research "Het Spelderholt"
Animal Sciences Group
Wageningen University and Research Centre
Netherlands

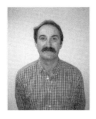

Greg B. Parkinson
Victorian Institute of Animal Science
475 Mickleham Road
Attwood
Victoria 5049
Australia

Contents

1

What is beak-trimming and why are birds trimmed?

Philip C. Glatz

Introduction

Beak-trimming is performed early in the life of commercial poultry to decrease injuries caused by the behavioural vices of cannibalism, bullying, feather and vent pecking and to avoid feed wastage. Beak-trimming is known to help flocks with a hysteria problem. Birds naturally peck at each other and their environment; this behaviour can become a problem in commercial situations (Glatz 2000).

Farm managers have their flocks beak-trimmed to blunt the beaks enough so that pecking cannot do any great damage. For the majority of birds beak-trimmed in the world today, it involves the partial removal of the upper and lower beak (Figure 1.1) using an electrically heated blade that cuts and cauterises the beak.

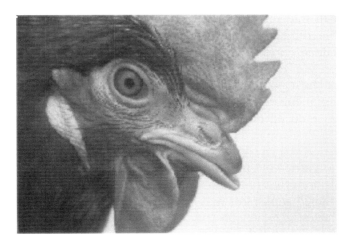

Figure 1.1 Beak-trimmed hen.

Without a correct beak-trimming program, the egg producer risks heavy losses of chickens and pullets from cannibalism and in the laying stage from protrusion and vent pick outs. In many cases these losses represent the major part of mortality. If birds are not trimmed, mortality of up to 25-30 % of the flock will occur and can be financially as disastrous as a disease outbreak (Glatz 2000).

New beak-trimming methods are being introduced into the industry. The infrared method directs a strong source of heat onto the inner tissue of the upper and lower beak. After a few weeks the tip of the upper and lower beak dies and drops off and the beak becomes shorter with blunt tips.

Beak-trimming is carried out at various ages depending on the preference of the farm manager. The most common ages for birds to be beak-trimmed are:

• Day old

• 5-10 days old

• 4-6 weeks old

• 8-12 weeks-of-age

• Touch up trim of adult birds (mainly in alternative systems)

The beak-trimmer holds the bird securely with its beak resting on a cutting bar. A foot pedal is then operated to bring the heated cutting blade down onto the beak. The blade cuts quickly and smoothly through the upper and lower beaks in one motion. The heat of the blade seals off the cut thus preventing bleeding and infection. Pain to the bird is reduced when the procedure is done correctly (Bourke, Glatz, Barnett and Critchley 2002).

Generally, the most popular age for beak-trimming is from 5 to 10 days-of-age. Trimming at this age results in fewer beak problems later in the birds' life as well as reduced mortality. Beak regrowth is also reduced (Bourke *et al.*, 2002).

Re-trimming is carried out if a birds' beak grows back enough to cause pecking damage. Birds are often re-trimmed at 8-12 weeks-of-age when this happens. Some non-trimmed adult birds may need trimming if pecking outbreaks occur.

Contract teams, individual farmers and some large poultry companies carry out beak-trimming. Contract teams trim the majority of birds.

History of beak-trimming

Debeaking has been a term used to describe the practice although the process does not remove the whole beak as the term debeaking implies. More recently scientists have used the term partial amputation instead of beak-trimming, although the beak does re-grow and receptors are functional in the regenerated beak tissue (Glatz, Lunam, Barnett and Jongman 1998).

Paring of the tip of the top beak (Kennard 1937; Robinson 1961) and beak burning were the first methods used by poultry farmers to control cannibalism in laying flocks. A gas torch was used by T. E. Wolfe in the San Diego county in California to burn off part of the upper beak of the hen and was very effective in controlling pecking vices especially feather pulling (Sundaresan and Jayaprasad 1979; Sundaresan, Jayaprasad and Kothandaraman 1979). Later a neighbour of Wolfe, W.K. Hopper, adapted a tinner's soldering iron by giving it a chisel edge, which enabled the operator to apply downward pressure on the upper beak to sear and cauterise the beak. The Lyon Electric Company took up some of these modifications, to develop the first beak-trimming machine. The Lyon Electric Company first brought out a heated knife attachment for a homemade beak support and frame. The name for the machine "debeaker" was coined in 1942 and registered in 1943.

Beak-trimming methods

Gas beak-trimming

This machine consists of a hot plate and cutting bar operated by means of a foot lever. The efficiency of the machine varies with gas pressure and wind conditions. Generally it is slow to use but is a useful portable machine for beak-trimming small numbers of birds (Pickett 1969). Producers can currently purchase a pocket style machine for trimming pullets which uses gas from a cigarette lighter as its heat source.

Electric soldering iron

Wilfred, Joseph and Jeganathan (1982) reported on a simple inexpensive device used for beak-trimming birds consisting of an ordinary electric soldering iron commonly used by a radio mechanic for soldering. A disk or coin made of brass or copper was welded to the tip of the soldering iron and the projecting edge of the circumference of the disc was sharpened like that of a blade. When the soldering iron was connected to the wall plug the temperature of the sharpened disc at the tip attains the maximum temperature (lead melting point 327°C) within a few minutes which is quite sufficient for cauterising the beak.

Hot blade machines

Following the development of the "debeaker" in 1943 there have been refinements to the machine including some control of cutting and cauterisation and control of blade temperature. However control of blade temperature is still assessed mostly by the colour of the blade, although thermocouples are available for measuring blade temperature. The most commonly used is the dark (dull) red heat with an approximate temperature of 650-750°C. Cherry red colour (850-950°C) is used for toe clipping.

The Lyon Electric Company in San Diego, California has been manufacturing hot blade beak-trimming machines for beak-trimming layers, broilers and turkeys for over 50 years. The Lyon Company (1982) suggest that precision beak-trimming of 6-10 day-old chicks is one of the most accurate methods available, using either the Super V precision beak-trimmer (Figure 1.2) or the Dual Debeaker. The machines have a timed cauterisation of 2 sec and Lyon suggests that properly done, this method of beak-trimming will suffice for the productive life of the bird. Both models of the debeaker are available in water-cooled and waterless models. Lyon also market a Super TT Debeaker which has been designed primarily for beak-trimming birds from 3-6 weeks-of-age, but can be used to trim beaks of birds up to 12 weeks-of-age, but proportionally less beak is removed at this age. With the TT method the bird is held sideways at a 90^0 angle to the blade. Both beaks are trimmed and cauterised simultaneously with an inward slant. Older bird beak-trimming is performed with the Super V debeaker but blades used for cutting are heavier. Lyon recommend that when birds are beak-trimmed up to 12 weeks-of-age, two-thirds of the upper beak is removed but no closer than 3.2 mm from the nostril. If the lower beak is trimmed it should protrude beyond the upper beak by 3.2 mm. Beak-trimming birds over 12 weeks is generally accomplished by removing the two-thirds to three quarters of the upper beak, again determined by the bird's age, and maintaining a distance of 3.2 mm from the nostril. This severity of beak-trimming is far greater than is allowed under the Code of Practice in some countries.

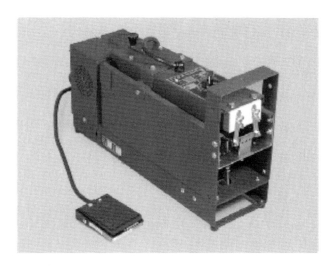

Figure 1.2 Lyon Super Debeaker (courtesy of Lyon Electric Co.)

Cold blade

Kennard (1937) was the first to use a method where the tip of the beak was separated from the deeper structures by traction or tearing. A short cut was made into one side of the beak only, extending into the margins about 1.5–3.2 mm (depending on the size of the beak) at a point 3.2–6.4 mm posterior to the tip. The flat side of the knife blade was placed against the cut portion of the beak and raised to loosen the edge. The tip was removed by applying traction toward the opposite side and down toward the lower mandible.

Peckham (1984) and Gleaves (1999) examined a temporary form of beak-trimming using a sharp jackknife. A nick is made in the beak about 6.4 mm from the tip, with the thumb holding the cut portion of the beak against the blade. The knife is rolled around the tip of the beak tearing off the horny portion and exposing the quick. If properly done there is little bleeding. It is not recommended to cut into the quick without cauterisation.

Grigor, Hughes and Gentle (1995) used a pair of secateurs at 1, 6 or 21 days to trim the upper beak of turkeys. There was bleeding from the upper mandible, which ceased shortly after the operation. Despite the beak regrowth a reduction of cannibalism was noted. Gleaves (1999) recommends the use of a dog nail clipper for trimming beaks to protect against the early cannibalism. Gentle (1997) and Gentle, Hughes, Fox and Waddington (1997) used secateurs to remove one-third of the upper beak in Isa Brown chickens.

There were very few differences observed between behaviour and production of the hot blade and cold blade trimmed chickens.

Robotic beak-trimming

Bock and Samberg (1990) reported information on the "Robot AG 4500" made by Gourlandt Industries Inc., Zoo-Techniquews, France which permits simultaneous automated beak-trimming and Marek's (sub cutaneous injection) and Newcastle-Bronchitis (eye drop) vaccination of day-old chicks. This equipment has the ability to treat up to 4,500 chickens per hour. While the AG 4500 is suitable for vaccination some problems emerged with the beak-trimming. The chicks were loaded onto the robot by hand being held by cups around their heads. If the chickens were not loaded correctly they could drop off the line, receive excessive beak-trimming or very light trimming because they were not positioned correctly on the holding cups. The machine could not beak-trim chickens effectively if there was a variation in the weight or size of chickens.

Chemical beak-trimming

Lunam and Glatz (1995a) reported on the use of capsaicin applied at the time of conventional hot blade beak-trimming to retard beak growth. Capsaicin is a cheap non toxic substance extracted from hot peppers. Applied topically or orally to mammals it induces a short term burning sensation. In contrast to this effect in mammals, capsaicin is reported to induce only mild behavioural responses when applied topically to birds (Mason and Maruniak 1983). Some bird species demonstrate a preference for food containing capsaicin. However, capsaicin does cause depletion of certain neuropeptides from sensory nerves in birds and thus may cause desensitisation as it does in mammals. Although its long term effect in birds is not known capsaicin can cause degeneration of sensory nerves in mammals. It is well known that if the nerve supply is removed or prevented from reinnervating a particular tissue, then the tissue will degenerate. Lunam and Glatz (1995a) showed that capsaicin decreases the rate of beak regrowth, and hence the need for re-trimming by its action on the sensory nerves, but operators must avoid contact with the substance during its application to the beak. The feeding ability of birds improved with capsaicin administration in the feed and therefore has the potential to reduce the percentage of starve-outs (Glatz 1990; Glatz and Lunam 1990).

Infrared beak treatment

Infrared Beak Treatment (IBT) is patented process developed by Nova-Tech Engineering of Willmar, Minnesota, USA. The Nova-Tech IBT system (Figure 1.3) is a bloodless procedure and uses a non-contact, high intensity, infrared energy source to treat beak tissue (Glatz 2004). The infrared heat source penetrates and treats the hard outer layer of the beak and treats the underlying basal tissue of the beak affecting the regeneration of the corneum. Initially, the corneum remains intact, protecting the treated soft basal layer tissue. Immediately following the process, the beak shows a whitening of the basal tissue and a white dot on the top of the beak, but the bird is able to continue to use its beak. Within a week the beak softens, and by two weeks after the treatment the sharp hook of the beak erodes away as the bird uses its beak. Because the infrared process initially affects mostly the basal tissue, a bird at four weeks-of-age will have a longer beak than a bird that has undergone a traditional beak cutting method. By twelve weeks-of-age, however, the infrared treated (Figure 1.4) beak will be shorter than the beak cut with the hot blade.

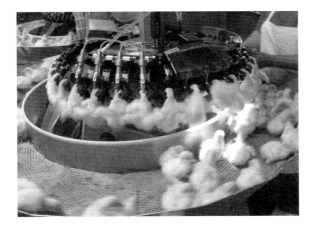

Figure 1.3 Infrared beak treatment machine (courtesy of Nova-Tech Engineering).

A head holding fixture (specific for turkeys, chickens and ducks) allows repeatability and accuracy. The head holder was generated from a mould of the specific species average size head. The entire front of the bird's cranium becomes the reference point to maintain repeatable treatment over a wide range of bird size. Birds with a larger cranium will reference the beak back farther versus smaller birds.

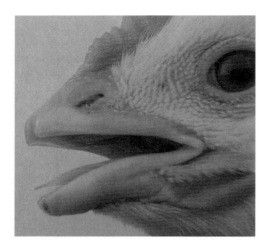

Figure 1.4 Infrared treatment of birds beaks (courtesy of Nova-Tech Engineering).

The amount of infrared energy applied to the beak is programmable, and variations in bird size due to flock age are accommodated. Each hatchery can set the treatment level to satisfy their customers' demands and expectations.

The IBT process is an integral part of the Poultry Services Processor (PSP). The system was designed to minimise the amount of bird handling, and administer several treatments after the bird is loaded. Currently a liquid injection and bird counter are available options. In the future, a nasal vaccination and the eye vaccination will be integrated into the standard PSP unit.

The PSP unit can only be leased and therefore requires no capital equipment costs. Nova-Tech Engineering installs and maintains the system for a lease rate. The PSP is divided into removable modules and is monitored via a communication system and on site computer. Machine malfunctions can be detected and diagnosed from facilities in the USA.

Laser machines

Lasers operate by sending energy to the target tissue, the heat is absorbed and in the process (if the beam is strongly directed) will result in cutting of the tissue. During the procedure there are intense emissions of light, each pulse lasting a fraction of a second on the area being treated. Many lasers are equipped with cooling systems to decrease temperature on the treated area, providing a mild anaesthetic effect. Human patients normally feel a burning or stinging sensation (Glatz 2004). Contour lasers are used in human medicine for surgical applications requiring the excision, incision, ablation, vaporisation and coagulation of tissue. The Yag lasers are used for hair and treatment of skin lesions. The lasers have an effective cooling system applied before, during and after each pulse, providing some prevention of pain.

In the carbon dioxide (CO_2) laser the pattern generator uses two galvanometers to rapidly steer the beam over a selected pattern (line, hexagon, diamond, square etc.) allowing areas of up to 1 cm^2 to be treated with precise control.

Laser beak-trimming

Rooijen and Haar (1997) reported on a laser method, which cut the beaks of day-old chickens with a laser beam. No details were provided by the authors on the type of laser used, or the severity of beak-trimming. By 16 weeks the beaks of laser trimmed birds resembled the un-trimmed beaks, but without the bill tip. Feather pecking and cannibalism during the laying period were highest among the laser trimmed hens. These results suggest that the severity of laser beak-trimming was insufficient, enabling regrowth of the beaks. It was expected that laser beak-trimming, would enable greater uniformity in beak-trimming and improve welfare.

Glatz (2004) reported on the use of an ophthalmic laser (1.5W; 4 sec pulse; 50-micron spot size) that successfully cut through an upper beak sample from a cull chicken. Two passes of the laser beam were required to complete the cut. There was insufficient power in the laser beam to cut the beak tissue in one action. Live bird studies with day-old chickens established the spot size to enable coagulation of the tissue and prevent bleeding. When a 50-micron spot size was used for 2 sec there was insufficient energy density of the laser beam on the tissue to cause coagulation and the beak began to bleed. The spot size was increased to 200 microns with a cutting time of 2 sec. The birds vocalised more in response to the increase in energy density indicating they were feeling more discomfort. There was no bleeding from the wound indicating that the 200-micron spot size was effective, not only in cutting the tissue, but also in sealing the wound. The laser was able to cut through the outer layers of keratin, but was not able to cut the inner bone. The lack of success in being able to cut the bony portion of the beak with an opthalmic laser was considered to be due to the lack of power. Subsequently a green laser and a CO_2 laser were tested. The CO_2 laser with a 1 sec pulse, 50-micron spot size and power rating of 10W was the most effective laser in cutting a beak sample. The experiments showed that there is potential to use lasers for beak-trimming and demonstrated the spot size required to cauterise the beak, and the power to cut the beak. Further work is now required to develop the design of a prototype laser beak-trimming machine with automatic measurement and laser trimming of the beak to the required standards.

Bio beak-trimming

The Bio-Beaker uses a high voltage electrical current to burn a small hole in the upper beak of chickens. In the 1980's the Bio-Beaker (Sterwin Laboratories, Millsboro, Delaware, USA) was developed which used a high voltage arc (1500 Volt AC electric current) across two electrodes to burn a small hole in the upper beak of chickens. Up to 2000 day-old chicks can be beak-trimmed in an hour using this process. The chicks being bio-beaked struggled as the beak is inserted into the mask of the instrument and also when the current is passed. Grigor *et al.* (1995) reports that it takes 0.25 sec to burn a hole in the beak. The primary advantage of the Bio-Beaker is that an adequate beak-trim is achieved during the first day of life, making the unit ideal for use in the hatchery. This allows treated chickens to eat and drink normally for the first few days with their beaks intact. It was originally hoped that after a period of 3-7 days the tip of the beak would die and slough off leaving a rounded stump. The aim was to burn a hole in the upper beak at a point just beyond the horny projection. In about 4 days the chick should begin to lose that portion of the upper beak from the hole to the tip and by 10-14 days-of-age, this portion of the beak should be completely lost from all the chickens.

Unfortunately in many chicks the tip of the beak did not slough off and birds had to be re-trimmed using conventional equipment. In turkeys, however, the Bio-Beaker was more successful (Grigor *et al.,* 1995) with the beak tip falling off in 5-7 days and the wound healed by 3 weeks (Noble and Kestor 1997). This method is used for trimming the upper beak of turkeys but operator errors and inconsistencies have caused welfare problems for turkeys. In this respect Renner, Nestor and Havenstein (1989) found that severe arc beak-trimming 1 mm from the nostril in turkeys increased mortality relative to hot blade trimming. In contrast Noble, Muir, Kruegar and Nestor (1994) compared arc trimming and intact beak males and found no difference in mortality of male turkeys.

Not unrelated to the bio-beak process was the method developed for broiler chickens by Smith (1997) who used the hot blade to burn an area near the tip of the upper beak. The procedure allowed a thin base to exist to the tip of the beak. The chick could eat and eventually the upper beak dropped off.

Freeze drying method

O'Malley (1999) used liquid nitrogen to declaw emus but found the conventional hot blade method was more effective. The freeze drying method was costly, time consuming and regrowth of the claws occurred. Development of equipment that could freeze and cut the beaks, however, may be worth investigating.

Cannibalism

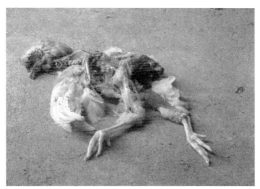

Figure 1.5 Cannibalised pullet (courtesy of M Choct).

The main purpose of beak-trimming is to prevent cannibalism (Figure 1.5), which occurs when birds peck at and consume the tissue of another bird (Allen and Perry 1975). An outbreak of cannibalism is easy to recognise. The main indicators are blood stained birds, broken skin, raw wounds and injured vents (Savory 1995). Cannibalism occurs in most strains of birds, at any age and in all production systems (Hughes and Duncan 1972; Kjaer, Rutter, Rushen, Randle and Eddison 1995; Klemm, Reiter and Pingel 1995). The incidence of cannibalism is greater in brown-egg layers compared to white-egg layers (Abrahamsson, Tauson and Elwinger 1996). Many causes of cannibalism have been suggested, but often outbreaks occur in one pen while similar environmental conditions or feeding practices in other pens on the same farm do not cause any difficulty. Cannibalism develops either as a result of misdirected ground pecking (Blokhuis 1986) or is associated with dust bathing behaviour (Vestergaard 1994; Johnsen, Vestergaard and Norgaard 1998). Other reports suggest that cannibalism occurs due to poor housing (Baum 1995), high stocking density (Savory 1995), large group size (Lee and Moss 1995), high light intensity (Kjaer and Vestergaard 1999), increasing day length (Nixey 1994), nutritional deficiencies (Esmail 1997; Savory, Mann and MacLeod 1999) and feed form (Bessei, Reiter, Bley and Zeep 1999).

Prolapse

Picking of the vent region or region of the abdomen several inches below the vent is the severest form of cannibalism (Allen and Perry 1975; Savory 1995). Predisposing conditions are prolapses or tearing of the tissues by passage of an abnormally large egg especially early in the laying cycle. Alternatively, pecking may be directed at the small downy feathers below the cloaca. After birds have tasted blood they will continue their cannibalistic habits without provocation. Smith (1982) suggested cannibalistic pecking is responsible for at least 80% of all prolapses and often results from poor beak-trimming with the offender usually being a bird that has been improperly beak-trimmed. The true prolapse is a condition that occurs during the first stages of lay when the pullet has suffered a rupture of the tissues of the lower part of the reproductive tract. Usually a prolapse occurs because of poor muscular elasticity or tone and may be the result of a hen laying too large an egg for its age. Prolapse occurs when fat pullets have been put into production, where pullets have been indirectly light stimulated or where flocks have not been reared uniformly and have under developed members.

Pecking

If a bird pecks itself and the feather or toes are damaged it is referred to as self pecking or self mutilation while pecking other birds is referred to as allo-pecking (Van Hierden, Korte, Ruesink, Van Reenen, Engel, Korte-Bouws, Koolhaas and Blokhuis 2002a). Aggressive pecking is forceful allo-pecking usually directed to the head (Kruijt 1964). Feathers can be damaged, with a strong correlation between severe pecks and feather damage (Bilcik and Keeling 1999). Caution needs to be exercised using plumage condition as an indicator of feather pecking as it can be confounded with abrasion. Often genetic variability in feather pecking is expressed at older ages only (Kjaer 2001). Feather pecking can be the precursor of cannibalism. Naked areas appear on the bird's body especially the back, tail and the vent which can lead to further pecking (McAdie and Keeling 2000). This is sometimes caused by feather mites or by moulting. Slow feathering strains are more susceptible to feather pecking. In its mildest form it has been observed as barb pecking. Mould growth and mycotoxins in feed can cause abnormal feathering contributing to feather pecking (Elliot 1995). Feather abnormalities have also been attributed to deficiencies of zinc, tryptophan, lysine, glycine, leucine, arginine, valine, isoleucine, phenylalanine and tyrosine (Elliot 1995). Dietary deficiencies of pantothenic acid, folic acid, vitamin B12, vitamin E, pyridoxine, and biotin also contribute to poor feathering. Van Hierden, Korte, Ruesink, Van Reenen, Engel, Korte-Bouws, Koolhaas and Blokhuis (2002b) reported that differences in feather pecking between a high feather pecking line and a low feather pecking line are associated with differences in andrenocortical activity, serotonin and dopamine turnover in the brain providing an explanation of the individuals vulnerability to exhibit pecking abnormalities.

Types of pecking

Feather pecking involves a hen approaching another hen from behind or from the side, focusing on the feathers of the other hen (Van Hierden *et al.*, 2002a). Initially the other hen pays no attention, but will move away after having received some pecks, the response depending on the severity of pecks. Pecking without removal of feathers usually causes little damage and can include barb pulling, barb pecking (Savory 1995), gentle pecking and stereotype pecking (Keeling 1995). Pecking which causes damage includes feather removal (resulting in damage to the integument including bleeding from follicles), feather pulling (Savory 1995) and severe pecking (Keeling 1995). Birds may be wounded by feather pecking or even pecked to death. Cannibalism can occur without previous feather pecking. This form is directed at the cloaca and is referred to as cloacal cannibalism or vent pecking (Hughes and Duncan 1972). Cloacal pecking is thought to be the precursor of cannibalism but high rates of feather pecking does increase the risk of cannibalism (Wechsler, Huber and Nsh 1998).

Feather pulling

Feather pulling is most frequently seen in flocks in close confinement. Nutritional and mineral deficiencies may be contributing factors. Sometimes the feather is removed and eaten. Irritation caused by lice and mites may induce this vice (Glatz 2000).

Feather eating

Pullets prefer to eat shorter filoplumes (<10 cm) and long feathers are eaten when short feathers are not available (McKeegan and Savory 1999). It has been suggested oil on the surface of the feathers originating from the preen gland may provide the olfactory cue. This is supported by observations that feathers around the preen gland are targeted when pecking damage takes place. Feather eating begins in the growing period following a moult at 9-11 weeks. The low availability of suitably sized moulted feathers from 16 weeks onwards may explain the increase in pecking damage. Monitoring floor feather availability in breeding programs could be a simple approach to suppress pecking problems (McKeegan, Savory, MacLeod and Mitchell 2001).

Toe picking

Toe picking is most commonly seen in domestic chicks and is often initiated by hunger or by excessive warmth (Seetha Rama Rao 1988). It is a particularly serious vice among young chicks reared on dark coloured litter and can lead to an increase in mortality and a reduction in growth. Strong light illuminates the blood in the quick of the toes attracting the attention of the other chicks. Toe picking is a current problem in hens housed in aviary systems in Europe.

Head picking

Head picking is directed by dominant birds at birds low in the pecking order causing the recipient to vocalise (Savory 1995). In severe cases the areas above the eyes are black and blue with sub cutaneous haemorrhage, wattles are dark and swollen and ear lobes are black and necrotic. Even though birds have trimmed beaks they will peck at a neighbouring hen or grasp its ear lobe or wattles and shake their heads in much the same fashion as a terrier shaking a rat. Wood-Gush (1959) reports on breeds of birds selected for fighting in Roman times with little systematic selection against this vice occurring since then. The modern bird's aggressive behaviour may be a legacy of this approach.

Cannibalism in alternative systems in Europe

Although free-range and barn systems enable the birds greater freedom to express natural behaviour, vices such as feather pecking, cannibalism and mislaid eggs continue to be a problem in alternative systems in Europe (Tauson and Abrahamsson 1992; Blokhuis and Metz 1996; Kathle and Kolstad 1996). Losses of up to 13% have been reported in an aviary (Hill 1986) and of up to 15% in both a strawyard (Gibson, Dun and Hughes 1988) and a free-range system (Keeling, Hughes and Dun 1988). Michie and Wilson (1985) did not beak-trim birds prior to housing in perchery but it was found necessary to beak-trim five of the six pens because of cannibalism. The presence of males has been an important factor in reducing this behaviour problem in females.

Cannibalism seems to be much worse in some aviary systems than in the same strain of birds kept in cages although the problem is not consistent. Under these circumstances (Norgaad-Nielsen, Kjaer and Simonsen 1993) suggests that it may be essential to beak-trim laying hens in alternative systems on welfare grounds. On the other hand Appleby and Hughes (1991) report that where flocks in alternative systems have been compared directly with cages and no cannibalism problems occurred mortality was similar. However when cannibalism did occur it was 14.6% in an aviary and 13.3% in a straw yard.

In Norway different aviaries, litter floor and free-range systems have been introduced but cannibalism is a problem in large flocks since beak-trimming is prohibited (Lervik, Oppermann Moe, Tauson, Hetland and Svihus 2001).

In Sweden where beak-trimming is banned, feather pecking and cannibalism in furnished small group cages on commercial farms is rare although medium heavy brown birds showed poorer plumage compared to most white hybrids. Some strains have been withdrawn from the market (Tauson and Holm 2001). Initial experience of birds (which are all beak-trimmed) in new furnished cages at Gleadthorpe in the UK indicate that despite some isolated feather pecking in specific cages, plumage condition has remain good (Walker and Elson 2001). In the Netherlands Fiks-van Niekerk (2001) reports that hens in large furnished cages (20 or more hens) that are not beak-trimmed tend to perform more feather pecking. Mortality was high (14.8-21.9%) in large furnished cages in some trials due to cannibalism. It was considered the lighting system caused the problems with feather pecking and cannibalism.

For organic poultry farming systems feather pecking and cannibalism is a problem (Fiks-van Niekerk 2001). A survey of Dutch organic farms with laying hens showed that 50% of the flocks have severe problems with cannibalism, 25% have moderate problems and only 25% have no or few problems with feather pecking (Bestman, 2000 reported by Fiks van-Niekerk, 2001). This is considered to be caused by the larger group sizes.

In Switzerland Hirt (2001) examined feather pecking on 12 aviary farms with outside runs. Problems with feather pecking increased as flock size increased from 50 to 3000 hens.

In the UK feather pecking and cannibalism are controlled where possible in free-range systems by trimming one-third of the beak at 10 days. This is only partly effective and unpredictable outbreaks of cannibalism still occur. This is reflected by the mean mortality levels being about 5% in cages and 8% in free range. If beak-trimming is not practised, mortality in free range is about 16%. A comparison of the management and husbandry of 112 free-range flocks in the UK revealed that feather pecking was greatest when a low percentage of the flock used the outside range. This has the result of increasing the stocking density within the house, which increases the bird to bird interactions (Nicol, Lewis, Poetzsch and Green 2001). The use of plastic slats in the house reduced risk of feather pecking. The Shaver bird had a low propensity to use the outside range area. Farmers were generally reluctant to try and increase range use, although they were receptive to other management changes, like litter condition, diet and reducing the use of bell-type drinkers (Green, Lewis, Kimpton and Nicol 2000).

There is always a chance of an outbreak of cannibalism in current alternative systems housing large flocks of laying hens. This is hampering the success of alternative housing systems that in principle possess great welfare advantages. No strategy guarantees that feather pecking will not develop in practical poultry keeping and beak-trimming may be required in specific cases to prevent the risk of welfare problems caused by cannibalism.

Conclusion

Beak-trimming of commercial layers is a common management practice used in the poultry industry to prevent feather pecking and cannibalism. Proper beak-trimming can result in greatly improved layer performance but improper beak-trimming can ruin an other wise good flock of hens. Re-trimming is practiced in most flocks, although there are some flocks that only need one trim. Hot blade beak-trimming is the most popular method and the method has remained unchanged for over 60 years. That is, a red-hot blade cuts and cauterises the beak. Sharp secateurs have also been used to trim the upper beak of both layers and turkeys but has not been used on a large scale in Industry. A robotic beak-trimming machine was developed in France, which permitted simultaneous, automated beak-trimming and vaccination of day-old chicks of up to 4500 chickens per hour but the method was not successful. A chemical method of beaktrimming using capsaicin was trialed and decreased the rate of beak regrowth by its action on the sensory nerves. It suffered the disadvantage of causing an extreme burning sensation in operators who come in contact with the substance during its application to the bird. More recently a laser method of trimming was tested but needs further development. The most promising new method is the infrared beak treatment system.

2

Ethics of beak-trimming and cannibalism

Neville G. Gregory

Introduction

In modern animal production, the ethical issues that are of greatest concern to the general public are:

- taking an animal's life

- surgery or mutilation without pain relief

- severe confinement

With each of these procedures there are three recurring questions:

- is it fair?

- is it necessary?

- are there alternatives?

In the case of beak-trimming, the separate issues run as follows:

Is beak-trimming fair on the animal?

- does it hurt? If so, is it a severe pain, and how long does the pain last?

- does beak-trimming compromise normal activities? In what ways are the beak-trimmed birds compromised and for how long?

- if it is applied badly, what are the consequences for the bird? Is improper application common?

Is beak-trimming necessary?

- is cannibalism inevitable when beak-trimming is not performed? If it is not inevitable, would cannibalism be common? How common?

- is the need for beak-trimming a sign of over-intensification in modern farming?

Are there alternative practices which avoid the need for beak-trimming?

- what are the alternatives?

- are those alternatives practical?

- do the alternatives impose any welfare compromises?

- are there any beak-trimming methods which are relatively painless or less compromising?

- does beak-trimming stop the cause of cannibalism?

Subsequent chapters in this book give answers to some of these questions, and the conclusions are as follows:

1.   beak-trimming hurts the birds when the beak is severely trimmed, and it is particularly painful for older birds.

2.   the pain is likely to be less if the beak is mildly trimmed, but is less effective at preventing cannibalism than a more extensive trim.

3.   severe beak-trimming affects the birds' ability to feed, drink, preen, explore and build nests. For example, there can be a period after beak-trimming when feed intake is reduced before the bird modifies its feeding and drinking methods.

4.   beak-trimming reduces the weapon that allows cannibalism, and it is usually effective in preventing or reducing cannibalism.

5.   at worst, the suffering associated with cannibalism is worse than the suffering associated with beak-trimming.

6.   when cannibalism occurs in un-trimmed flocks, it can lead to substantial mortality and culling (up to 30% of the flock), and the enterprise becomes less economic.

7.   cannibalism is not inevitable in untrimmed birds. It depends on bird temperament, competition for resources, ambient lighting, group size, social structure, hormonal status, hunger, and stocking density. The Brambell Committee (1965) put some emphasis on the fact that

cannibalism is seldom a problem when the victims can take appropriate avoidance action and they have room to get away from bullies. However, modern egg production systems involve large numbers of birds stocked at densities that allow a useful level of production, and successful avoidance behaviour is not always possible.

8.   it is not known how common cannibalism would be if all flocks, both loose-housed and caged, were not beak-trimmed. However, it is appreciated that cannibalism would be more common in warm climates where birds are housed in open-sided sheds which have stronger lighting levels.

9.   when badly applied, beak-trimming has been known to cause mouth blisters, bulbous deformities at the severed end of the beak, tongue damage and burnt nostrils.

10.   the alternatives to beak-trimming for avoiding cannibalism include selecting docile strains, controlling light intensity, providing alternative pecking substrates, providing adequate room for birds to escape when harassed, removing sick or victimised birds and culling them or managing them separately, ensuring that there is an adequate feed supply, and avoiding abrupt changes in feed.

11.   the alternatives to beak-trimming in managing an outbreak of cannibalism include reducing light intensity, scatter feeding a crumb, pellet or other feed source which provides alternative items to peck at, modifying the colour of the lighting, culling cannibalistic and victimised birds, and applying deterrents to the birds' plumage.

12.   many of the alternatives listed above would be feasible for particular situations. However, with the possible exception of genetic selection, none of them seem to be as effective as beak-trimming. Beak-trimming does not always produce lasting effectiveness, and in most flocks it has to be repeated.

13.   there are beak-trimming methods that cause less pain than others.

This level of technical detail does not, however, satisfy everyone. Some people take the view that all mutilations are unacceptable, and the need for performing a mutilation is an indictment on modern farming. It is argued that the poultry industry should not have to resort to beak-trimming to correct for frustration, aggression, unappeased hunger or whatever causes the birds to become cannibalistic in a particular situation.

An alternative outlook is that many species are cannibalistic, and it is a harsh reality that animals kill and eat their own kind even in the absence of pressures from mankind. It is worth digressing to compare cannibalism in different species.

Cannibalism in the animal kingdom

Cannibalism or infanticide occurs in chickens, turkeys, pigs, hyenas, ferrets, hamsters, mice, gerbils and a number of invertebrate species. It is particularly common amongst gastropods. In the case of the aquatic prosobranch *Natica unifasciata* the adult normally catches its prey by following scent trails or by tracing vibrations through the bed. On contacting the prey, which includes juveniles of its own species, it envelops the animal, and covers it with slime. The trapped prey is then towed to a sandy site where the *Natica* buries itself and its victim, before drilling through the shell and ingesting the contents. The European land snail (*Aegopinella nitidula*) attacks other land snails as well as juveniles of its own species through an aperture it rasps in the shell. Land snails are sensitive to potentially painful stimuli in the foot (Kavaliers, Hirst and Teskey 1983) and so it can be argued that the victim suffers, assuming that the saliva or slime of the *Aegopinella* does not have an analgesic effect.

The speed of the kill is all-important in determining the extent of suffering. In pigs, the sow bites the piglet through the head. Piglets that have been rescued from this situation had depressed fractures of the skull, and teeth marks on the jaws or neck. It should be a relatively humane death provided the sow or gilt completes the process promptly. Female Golden hamsters attack their victims with a spring in the air followed by a series of bites, usually directed at the head. This is similar to fighting behaviour seen between adults, and it can be provoked by a pup attempting to suckle a non-lactating female (Richards 1966). Whereas gerbils do not attack the pups. Instead they eat them in a normal manner. The pup is picked up in the mouth, carried to a corner, held in the forepaws, and eaten much as if it was a piece of food. The interval between first approach and the first bite is usually 15 to 25 sec.

In spotted hyenas infanticide occurs when marauding males kill pups, which they attack at the throat. In mice, death by infanticide is also very quick, and it is also the male which attacks the pups. This has been related to testosterone production. Castration of male mice reduces pup killing, and giving virgin female mice testosterone induces pup killing (Berryman 1986). Wild mice are more prone to infanticide than laboratory strains when kept in confinement, and environmental noise can provoke infanticide (Busnel and Molin 1978).

In chickens, turkeys and ducks, the time to unconsciousness and death during cannibalism is relatively long because the victims are often attacked on the back or rear end instead of the head or neck. This means that the potential duration of suffering is longer in poultry compared with other vertebrates. It may be closer to the situation seen with invertebrates. On this basis it is implicit that greater effort should be taken in preventing suffering during cannibalism in birds, when it is preventable.

Stocking density and cannibalism

The role that stocking density has in causing cannibalism needs special consideration. Firstly, it implies that poultry production has become too intensive for the type of animal being farmed. Secondly, stocking density has assumed political importance in animal welfare debates, and cannibalism is a key feature in these arguments.

When personal space is encroached, the animals may either move apart or threaten each other. Gregarious animals often adopt submissive behaviour when avoiding these threats, rather than flight behaviour. They may also show appeasement behaviour, which allows them to enter the personal space of a dominant animal without provoking a fight. Social species that have a strong aggressive drive, are more likely to attack and kill each other when personal space is invaded and they are kept in over-crowded conditions. This type of reaction can occur in carnivores, monkeys, rodents and birds, and in some situations there is an explosive outburst of aggression in what appeared to be an otherwise harmonious group.

Overcrowding places stress on animals because they are repeatedly encroaching on each others personal space (McBride 1971). Avoidance is impossible in this situation, and there is chronic stress. The dominant individuals may have greater freedom of movement, but the subordinates continuously direct their attention toward the dominant neighbour.

Often the overall space provided for animals is adequate to avoid this type of stress, but there can be localised crowding at the feeders, drinkers or other specific facilities. There needs to be sufficient space to avoid squabbling and intimidation.

The present recommendation for the maximum hen stocking density on deep litter is based partly on work which examined the space needed to perform normal static activities such as wing stretching, wing flapping, preening and feather fluffing (Baxter 1994). From that work it is thought that hens should be provided not less than 1425 cm^2/bird. This space is shown in Figure 2.1, and it equals 7 birds/m^2. While this may appear to provide sufficient area to perform static activities, the real space requirement necessary to limit aggression may be more than this.

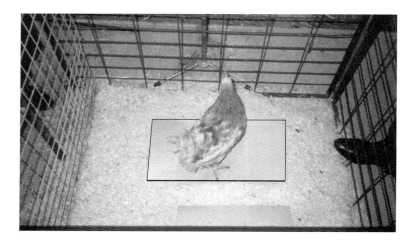

Figure 2.1 Layer hen standing on a piece of paper which is 1425 sq.cm.

There is very little aggression at low stocking densities where hens have a lot of space, and at high stocking densities if they are confined. It is highest at intermediate densities (Polley, Craig and Bhagwat 1974; Hughes and Wood-Gush 1977). The reduced aggression at very low densities may be due to greater opportunity to escape other hens. The reduced aggression at high densities may be due to one of two factors:

- the close presence of a dominant bird which prevents aggression between subordinates.

- aggression may be triggered by entry into the personal space rather than constant presence in the personal space.

In hens, cannibalism is more common in loose-housed alternative systems than in cage systems, probably because once it starts it can spread more easily throughout the whole flock. In addition, the small group size in conventional cages allows the development of a stable hierarchy. This does not mean to say that cannibalism cannot be controlled in alternative systems, but, it needs more focused management.

During the late 1980's a number of caged layer farms in the UK converted to perchery systems. The cages were removed from the sheds and in their place, wooden perching frames, wooden nestboxes and either slatted floors or litter and slatted floors were installed. At some units, the hens were stocked at over 25 birds/m². From experience it was found that these stocking densities were too high. The birds were dirty, from being fouled by other birds higher in the perching frame, and some farms experienced uncontrollable outbreaks of cannibalism.

Practical and research experience also indicates that the prevalence of cannibalism may vary between different types of alternative system.   For example, in the UK, some of the worst cases of cannibalism during the early 1990's occurred in high level percheries. This was supported by research at Gleadthorpe Farm in the UK where five systems were compared under controlled conditions within the same building. The high level perchery, which was stocked at the highest density, resulted in the greatest prevalence of cannibalism (Table 2:1).

Table 2.1 Prevalence of cannibalism in three trials of loose-housed layer hens.

System	Prevalence of cannibalism (%)
Free range	5.2
Deep litter	12.7
Aviary	14.1
Wood & wire	17.2
Wood/wire & litter	17.4
Conventional cage	9.2
Colony cage	14.3
Tiered wire floor	4
Low level perchery	4
High level perchery	16
Litter & wire floor	10
Conventional cage	1
Conventional cage	1.3
Marielund	3.1
Tiered wire floor	11.0
Voleatage	4.9

Cannibalism and cruelty

Failure to prevent or control cannibalism in farmed animals could be considered cruel. Cruelty comes in four forms, according to its cause (Gregory 1998a). It can be due to:

- Ignorance

- Inexperience

- Incompetence

- Inconsideration

When cannibalism gets out of hand, it is usually due to ignorance or inexperience on the part of the stockperson. Cannibalism is usually controllable, if there is adequate vigilance and prompt reaction, which may involve beak-trimming. However, if flock sizes become larger in the future, it will be less feasible to use beak-trimming as a method for controlling an outbreak. The practicality of beak-trimming 25,000 hens in a flock would be daunting, and instead there will be greater dependence on reducing lighting. In some situations training and familiarisation with how to recognise the early signs of cannibalism, and how to manage an outbreak, could be beneficial.

Conclusions

The ethical questions that need to be asked about beak-trimming are: is it fair, is it necessary and are there alternatives? The poultry industry usually argues that beak-trimming is fair, because the consequences to the birds of cannibalism in untrimmed flocks are appalling. For this reason, many members of the industry would claim that it is a necessary procedure. This claim is made even though there is a poor understanding of the prevalence and risk of cannibalism in untrimmed birds maintained in otherwise well-managed situations. There are alternatives to beak-trimming but so far they have not been as effective or reliable as beak-trimming. The counter-arguments against beak-trimming are based largely on an ideology which states that modern farming should not need to resort to mutilations in order to correct for over-intensification. It is claimed that high stocking densities are a particularly important factor leading to cannibalism. There is also the view that applying a painful procedure to all birds in order to correct a condition that may only arise in a minority is unacceptable.

We should not forget that cannibalism occurs in feral animals as well as farmed species such as poultry. However, this does not absolve the poultry industry from striving to manage and prevent cannibalism. In fact, death from cannibalism in poultry is likely to incur longer-lasting suffering than is the case for feral species, and so control of cannibalism in poultry has a stronger imperative. Failure to control cannibalism in farmed poultry verges on cruelty.

One approach used in teaching Applied Ethics in Agriculture is to apply the SOCLAP principle (Gregory 1998b). It allows one to consider an issue from every perspective. It does not tell one what to think, but it is helpful in telling one how to think. SOCLAP is an acronym for all the responsibilities or interests that are involved in an issue. It stands for:

- Society

- Oneself

- Customer or client

- Legal

- Animal

- Profession

Society's view is one step removed from the reality of farming. It usually leans towards indifference, or towards an idealised situation. The majority of society would probably not hold a view on beak-trimming, but when pressed it would consider that trimming should not be used, and there would be division as to whether it must not be used.

Oneself - do you feel comfortable with beak-trimming? Is this based on practical experience or a full knowledge of the procedure and its consequences?

Customer or client - what position do retailers and restaurant owners hold on beak-trimming? The signs are that their views could reflect the more sensitive concerns that society holds, in which case they would disfavour the continuation of beak-trimming.

Legal - legislation is intended to meet the needs of each nation. The needs will vary between countries, and it will be difficult to achieve harmonisation on farming issues such as beak-trimming where there are substantial differences in commercial investment. In many countries there is pressure on Governments from Animal Welfare pressure groups to phase out beak-trimming. Some Governments are now taking a less tolerant or reactive attitude towards such pressure, because they feel they are being lobbied and manipulated by an undemocratic process. When legislation is drafted, expert panels usually advise the Minister who in turn is responsible for making decisions and is accountable within the democratic process. In some countries the expert panels are only required to examine the animal welfare issues, whereas in others they have a broader remit and a stronger commercial focus.

Animal - the animal's best interests are no beak-trimming and no cannibalism. Beak-trimming is the lesser of the two insults, but it applies to all birds, whereas cannibalism would be sporadic in flocks that are not trimmed.

Table 2.2 Comparison of the advantages and disadvantages of beak-trimming in poultry.

Advantages	Disadvantages
Relatively effective in reducing the risk of cannibalism	Causes acute pain
Can be used to control an outbreak of cannibalism in small flocks	Can result in long term pain
Can be associated with improved feed conversion efficiency through reduced feed wastage	Reduced ability to sense materials with the beak or bill
May help reduce fearfulness in the flock because dominant birds have reduced beaks	Temporary debilitation, until the bird learns ways of using its shorter beak or bill
	Reduced ability to feed, drink, preen, explore and build nests until the bird learns to adapt to its reduced beak
	Difficult to apply in large loose-housed flocks when there is an outbreak of cannibalism
	Unsightly, especially when there is sizzling during the burning and bleeding afterwards

Profession - the majority of the poultry industry accepts beak-trimming as a necessary procedure. It would be happy not to have to trim the beaks of the chicks if there was a satisfactory alternative, but presently the threat of cannibalism from not beak-trimming is too serious to discontinue the practice without a satisfactory alternative.   Beak-trimming is a relatively simple solution for a problem that is difficult to predict. A minority within the industry consider that beak-trimming is unacceptable or unnecessary for their farming conditions.

The advantages and disadvantages of beak-trimming as a method for controlling cannibalism are listed in Table 2.2. Presently it serves a purpose, but because of the ethical concerns and welfare compromises it imposes, the general consensus is that it should be replaced with a more appropriate alternative method. The development of a better alternative should be a priority for the poultry industry, Governments and Animal Welfare pressure groups.

3

Acute and chronic pain in beak-trimmed chickens

Heng-wei Cheng

Introduction

A bird's beak is a complex, functional organ with an extensive nerve supply and various sensory receptors (Gentle and Breward 1981; Breward 1983; Gentle and Breward 1986; Gentle 1989; Megret, Rudeaux, Faure and Picard 1996). Beak-trimming may lead to pain (acute, chronic, or both) due to tissue damage and nerve injury.

Pain and pain regulation systems

Pain in humans is defined as an unpleasant sensory and emotional experience associated with actual or potential tissue damage (Merskey and Bogduk 1994). A similar definition of pain also applies to animals: pain is an aversive sensory and emotional experience by the animal in response to damage or a threat to the integrity of its tissues (Molony and Kent 1997). In animals, as in humans, pain has both a physiological sensory and a psychological or emotional component, but pain in animals is relatively difficult to recognize and assess since the exact nature of the emotional component remains uncertain (Wall 1992; Anil, Anil and Deen 2002), and an animal is unable to report the qualitative and quantitative dimensions of the sensory (pain) and emotional experience.

Pain is usually elicited by the activation of specific nociceptors (the Latin *nocere*, "to hurt", nociceptive pain) or by damage to sensory nerve fibers (neuropathic pain), resulting from inflammation and injury such as beak-trimming in birds. Most nociceptors, i.e. free unmyelinated nerve endings, are selective in their response to stimuli, but many nociceptors (polymodal nociceptors) respond to mechanical, thermal, and chemical stimuli. Nerve signals arising from activated nociceptors within the sites of tissue and nerve injury are transferred to the surface layers (lamina I and II) and the neck (lamina V) of the dorsal horn of the spinal cord by lightly myelinated (Aδ) and unmyelinated (C) fibers (Figure 3.1, Table 3.1); the signals then ascend to the thalamus through the spinothalamic tract, mediating the discriminative component of pain sensation and, together with the spinoreticular tract, produce the emotional-affective component of pain sensation (Mense 1983). Based on Melzack and Wall's "Gate Control Theory" of pain (Melzack and Wall 1965), the nociceptive system undergoes modulation at the dorsal horn level of the spinal cord. Pathological activities of sensitized nociceptors lead to plastic alterations at both peripheral and central levels following an injury or inflammation. These changes increase peripheral sensitization and central hyperexcitability and reduce inhibitory interneuron tone in the dorsal horn, leading to a decrease in the pain threshold and hyperalgesia (increase in the intensity of pain) as well as allodynia (pain elicited via activation of normally non-painful Aβ fibers (Millan 1999) by a non noxious stimulus such as touch (Table 3.1).

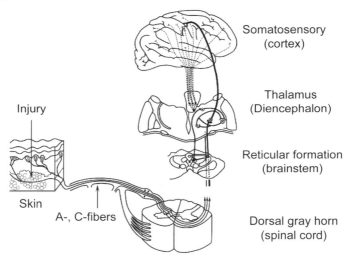

Figure 3.1 Diagrammatic representation of an injury on the skin leading to transmission in the nociceptive pathways, resulting in pain and hyperalgesia. (The figure was modified from Figure 12.28, In: Neuroscience, edited by Bear, M.F., Connors, B.W. and Paradiso, M.A., 2001).

Although animals including birds have a less developed cortex as compared to humans, both share similar subcortical structures and functions in response to painful stimuli (Iggo 1984; Zayan 1986; Sommerhoff 1990). The differences in the neuroanatomy among species represent neurological variations rather than differences in pain sensation. Many similarities in pain-induced behavioral and physiological responses have been found between humans and animals (Anil *et al.*, 2002). In addition, analgesics are effective in reducing pain in both humans and animals (Nolen 2001; Paul-Murphy

Table 3.1 Comparative properties of primary afferent fibers.

Type	Morphological features	Physiological features — Threshold for activation	Principal transmitters	Sensation mediated — Physiological features	Sensation mediated — Pathological features
C	0.4-1.2 um in diameter; Unmyelinated	slow conduction	SP/NKA; CGRP; EAA	Noxious (pain)	Highly noxious (hyperalgesia) Cold allodynia (pain)
Aδ	2-6 um in diameter; Lightly myelinated	intermediate velocity	SP/NKA; CGRP; EAA	Noxious (pain)	Highly noxious (hyperalgesia) Cold allodynia (pain)
Aß	> 10 um in diameter	fast velocity	EAA	Innocuous (no pain)	Mechanical allodynia (pain) Myelinated

EAA = Excitatory amino acid; CGRP = Calcitonin-gene related peptide; NKA = Neurokinin A; SP = substance P.

and Ludders 2001), which suggests that animals, at least among vertebrates, appear to have nociceptive pathways that conduct pain in a similar manner (Smith and Boyd 1991; Carstens and Moberg 2000; Underwood 2002). In application of these results, it indicates that procedures that cause pain in humans should also be considered to cause pain in animals (Interagency Research Animal Committee 1985; Carstens and Moberg 2000; Stokes 2000; Lee 2002), but animal and human pain may not be the same (Bateson 1991; Molony 1992). The more complex, integrated pain reactions vary across and within species and individuals (Underwood 2002; Stasiak, Maul, French, Hellyer and VandeWoude 2003). When assessing pain, a distinction should be made between what an animal may feel and what a human observing the animal may feel (Sanford, Ewbank, Molony, Tavernor and Uvarov 1986). Assessing pain in animals is also influenced by multiple factors, including species, breed, genetic strain, age, sex, and production status; the animal's experiences such as pain-related problems, the type of inflammation and lesion and lesion size; and its environments, such as stocking density (group size), cage or pen size, and food and water supplies. A combined investigation of behaviour, physiology, immunity, and neuroendocrinology should be considered when evaluating pain in animals.

Pain induced by beak-trimming

A bird's beak is a complex, functional organ with an extensive nerve supply (Gentle and Breward 1981; Breward 1983; Gentle and Breward 1986; Gentle 1989; Megret *et al.*, 1996). Following beak-trimming, several anatomical, physiological, and biochemical changes occur in cut peripheral nerves and damaged tissues. In the peripheral nervous system, injured nerves send out sprouts, which form neuromas, causing spontaneous activity and increased sensitivity to mechanical stimuli and various internal and external neurochemicals (Wall 1983; Devor 1994; Chen, Cohen and Hallett 2002). In the damaged tissue, lesion-induced inflammation releases algesic chemicals, which in turn depolarize the nociceptors of the nerve fibers, resulting in sensitization in both the peripheral and central nervous system (Carstens 1995; Millan 1999; Zimmermann 2001). Both peripheral and central sensitizations cause great responses to stimuli and lead to pain that develops over time in trimmed birds. Physiological and behavioural evidence reveals that pain and heightened beak sensitivity persist for several weeks or months following beak-trimming. In animals, following an injury or damage, pain reactions can be divided into three phases: painless, acute pain, and chronic pain (Table 3.2), which share a similar sequence of pain phases as found in humans post injuries.

Table 3.2 A general pathophysiological classification of phases and some major characteristics of pain.

Type (phases)	Duration	Temporal features relationship to cause	Major characteristics	Class	Source of pain	Adaptive response
Painless	Hours	Immediately follows an injury	"Similar to normal"			
Acute pain	Seconds to	Instantaneous; simultaneous	"Proportional to cause" withdrawal or escape		Principally nociceptive	Transient nociceptor
	Days	Resolves upon recovery	Hyperalgesia; allodynia spontaneous activity	Neuropathic	Plasticity of nerve systems	Quiescence; avoidance of contact with injured tissues
Chronic pain	Weeks to months	Persistent Exceed resolution of tissue damage	Hyperalgesia; allodynia; spontaneous pain; verbal pain and affective components	Neuropathic	Plasticity of the peripheral and central nervous systems	Physical, physiological, psychological and cognitive damage

Painless phase

The painless phase immediately following an injury is more common than has previously been recognized in both humans and animals, especially in circumstances where high priority behaviors are present, such as fighting and escaping (Wall 1979; Schott 2001). Pain also occurs very late in the case of sudden injury (Wall 1979), such as following beak-trimming that leads to sudden damage of a bird's beak. A pain-free period in trimmed birds lasts at least several hours and could be longer than 24 hours post beak-trimming (Gentle 1991). The painless period was verified behaviorally. Numbers of pecking in trimmed birds did not change at 6 h and dropped at 26 h post trimming. Recordings of electrical activity directly from the trigeminal nerve innervating the receptive fields near the site of cautery showed that there were no abnormal, spontaneously active units from 90 to 270 min post-beak-trimming, even though there was a massive injury discharge that lasted from 2 to 48 sec immediately following the procedure (Gentle 1991).

The painless phase immediately following beak-trimming may be related to a number of changes at both the peripheral and central nervous systems following the sudden lack of normal afferent inputs, including 1) injured nerves (shock and burn) temporally incapable of transmitting messages centrally from the injured region; 2) the biophysical continuity of the axoplasm with the extracellular milieu temporally sealed, and the acutely injured axons falling silent; 3) the message from activated large mechanoreceptive axons activating the interneurons which in turn suppress nociceptive signals to be transmitted to the central nervous system; and 4) analgesia due to released opioid peptides, a composition of the "endogenous analgesia system," from activated immune cells migrating directly to inflamed tissue, which subsequently occupy receptors localized on peripheral sensory nerves and result in antinociception (Wall 1979; Burchiel and Ochoa 1991; Schafer, Carter and Stein 1994; Cabot 2001; Schott 2001; Mousa 2003; Walker 2003).

Acute pain phase

The acute pain phase is a transition between coping with the cause of the injury and preparation for recovery, which could last a few minutes, hours, or days and should not outlast the healing process (Molony and Kent 1997). Acute pain is normally elicited by noxious stimulation of nociceptors, resulting from tissue damage or nerve injury. Activated nociceptors, i.e., a reduced pain threshold, increased pain sensitivity, or even spontaneous pain, provide signals to the central nerve system and trigger pain, resulting in hyperalgesia. Primary hyperalgesia conducted by activated C and Aδ nerve fibers occurs within the damaged tissue area, and secondary hyperalgesia which is conducted by activated mechanoreceptive Aß nerve fibers normally excited by innoxious stimulation, occurs in the tissue surrounding a damaged area, where it becomes supersensitive to stimulation, such as light and touch (Campbell, Raja, Meyer and Mankinnon 1988).

In humans and rodents, hyperalgesia is induced by inflammatory and neural changes following tissue damage or nerve injury. Damaged cells at the site of injury release a number of substances ("inflammatory soup") that bind to and open ion channels on nociceptor membranes, resulting in depolarizing and generating action potentials that convey the "pain message" to the central nervous system. The "inflammatory soup" consists of multiple mediators, such as bradykinin, adenosine triphosphate (ATP) and prostaglandins released from inflamed tissue, histamine from mast cells, cytokines including interleukin (IL)-1, IL-6, and tumor necrosis factor-alpha (TNF-α) from immune cells, and neurotransmitters including substance P and calcitonin-gene related peptide from injured nerve terminals (Figure 3:2) (Frisen, Risling and Fried 1993; Treede 1995; Tal 1999; Arruda, Sweitzer, Rutkowski and DeLeo 2000; McHugh and McHugh 2000; Cabot 2001; Jacques and Magali 2001; Homma, Brull and Zhang 2002; Cunha and Ferreira 2003; Schafer 2003). These pain-active factors act synergistically to increase sensitivity in the nociceptors and increase impulses of sensory afferent fibers. Pain-related changes in behaviour and physiology have been found in injured humans and animals, such as arousal, agitation, and aggressiveness or reduced locomotor activity as well as changes in eating and sleeping patterns. These changes can be inhibited by local anesthesia such as morphine and non-steroidal anti-inflammatory drugs including aspirin, which change pain mediators and produce pain relief mainly by restoring nociceptive sensitivity to its resting state.

Similar cellular mechanisms have been proposed for pain in beak-trimmed birds. Tissue and nerve damage caused by beak-trimming leads to a fast, early, but short-lasting increase in afferent nociceptive input, which is related to the first (primary) hyperalgesia. Due to the inflammatory reaction to tissue damage, sensitization occurs in the nociceptive transducers at the distal portion of beak stump, which in turn leads to a second wave of longer-lasting, afferent transmission of nociceptive impulses to the central nervous system and causes central hyperexcitability. The complexity of the encoding mechanisms transmits the tissue injury into the behavioral and physiological sequels associated with pain. Abnormal patterns of neural discharge have been revealed in the beak stump and could possibly cause acute pain (Breward

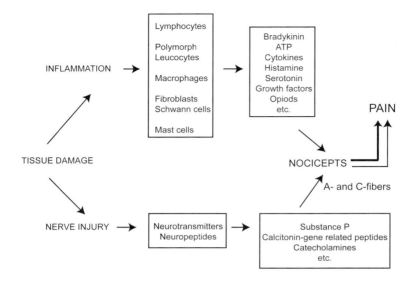

Figure 3.2 Diagrammatic representation of various mediators of pain ("inflammatory soup") produced by tissue damage and nerve injury.

1983; Breward 1985; Gentle 1986a). A similar, increased activity in nociceptors was recorded directly in the testes and tail of lambs post castration and tail docking (Molony and Kent 1997) and in the nerves of conscious humans who have reported that the stimulation was painful (Rice and Casale 1994). Beak-trimmed birds also showed an increase in heart rate (Glatz 1987) and a reduction of locomotor activity and sickness behavior, including loss of social behaviour, decrease in grooming, pecking, and movement, loss of appetite, and increased sleep duration (McIntosh, Slinger, Sibbald and Ashton 1962; Slinger, Pepper and Sibbald 1962; Eskeland 1981; Gentle, Hughes and Hubrecht 1982; Gentle 1986a; Gentle 1986b; Duncan, Slee, Seawright and Breward 1989; Craig and Lee 1990). Exhibition of these behaviors have been identified as reliable indicators of painfulness with lesion-induced sensitization of peripheral nociceptors in both humans and animals. Pain sensation can be relieved by analgesics. Compared to untreated birds, birds treated topically with analgesics (bupivicaine or isobutalone) had higher feeding rates (g of feed consumed divided by the time spent pecking at the food) post beak-trimming (Glatz, Murphy and Preston 1990), which indicated that pain-related reductions in pecking and eating had been overcome in the analgesic-treated birds. These results indicate that without effective interventions, beak-trimming induced hyperalgesia and allodynia could lead to pain and may likely cause chronic pain.

Chronic pain phase

The chronic pain phase is defined as an intense pain lasting weeks or months beyond the expected injury healing time (Molony and Kent 1997), or as pain involving an alteration in the nervous system that is capable of maintaining a painful state after the stimulus is removed and the injury is healed. Various hypotheses have been proposed to account for the hyperalgesia and spontaneous pain seen in humans and animal models of peripheral neuropathy. One of the most accepted hypotheses is that nerve injury or inflammation induces phenotypic changes predominantly in myelinated afferents. These changes cause a redistribution of membrane-bound ion channels, predominantly sodium channels, which lead to ectopic activity and spontaneous discharge of nociceptors and dorsal horn neurons, resulting in changes in the functions and structures of the peripheral and central nervous systems and causing peripheral and central sensitization.

Peripheral sensitization (peripheral hyperexcitability) is related to plasticity of nociceptive characteristics and formation of neuromas. The plasticity of nociceptors causes an increase in both sensation and the receptive field at and surrounding the injured sites and an activation of silent nociceptors. As much as 40% of C fibers and 30% of Aδ fibers are silent nociceptors, which can be activated only after inflammation or tissue damage. Activated silent nociceptors may develop a background discharge which is one of the cellular correlates of spontaneous pain. For example, in sciatic nerve-damaged rats, the post discharge in response to stimuli, particularly to a noxious pinch, was markedly greater in both magnitude and duration (Pitcher and Henry 2000), which correlates to hyperalgesia (nociceptive pain). Following a brief electrical stimulation of C-fibers, thermal hyperalgesia can develop rapidly and last 3 to 5 weeks (Vatine, Argov and Seltzer 1998). The peripheral sensitization and spontaneous pain could also be related to formation of neuromas in the proximal stump at the injured nerve fibers in the lesion site. A neuroma is a tangled mass of a terminal swelling or an endbulb sprouting from the proximal ending of a cut axon in the injured area. The sprouting can occur within 24 h of injury. In a neuroma, all sprouts are unmyelinated to begin with and, later, about 90% of all fibers are A-fibers. The neuroma is a source of substantial ectopic firing and triggers pain in humans and animals (Holland and Robinson 1990; Coderre, Katz, Vaccarino and Melzack 1993; Devor 1999; Devor and Seltzer 1999).

Central hyperalgesia (neuropathic pain) results as a consequence of certain events: the afferent inputs from increased excitability of nociceptors generated by injury and intense noxious stimuli enter the spinal cord, resulting in a pathological activation of central nociceptive neurons, which in turn leads to an anatomical reorganization of the central nociceptive neurons (chemical, structural, and functional plasticity), including a reduction of inhibitory interneuron tone (central hyperexcitability) in the dorsal horn of spinal cord (Baron 2000). These changes increase the receptive field and sensitivity of dorsal horn neurons to further stimulation (increases in central excitability). With regard to mechanical stimulation-evoked nociceptive neurons, the signals (either electric or chemical) released from those activated neurons play a critical role for both initiation and maintenance of nociceptive inputs leading to exaggerated responses to painful stimuli (hyperalgesia), producing neuropathic pain (Sheen and Chung 1993; Ji and Woolfe 2001).

Hypersensitivity can be investigated through quantitative sensory tests. For instance, hypersensitivity is detected when sensory stimulation evokes pain at stimulus intensities that do not induce pain in normal subjects. In other words, innocuous sensory stimulation or minimal nociceptive stimulation of peripheral tissues would be able to evoke exaggerated pain. Pain has been evidenced as changes in behaviors, such as guarding behaviour, i.e., relative inactivity, increase in sleep, decrease in eating and grooming, and social behavior disturbances, which prevent further injury.

Beak-trimming leads to tissue and nerve damage. The density of large myelinated fibers was reduced and the number of smaller myelinated fibers was increased in the beak stumps of birds trimmed at hatch, 8 days, or 6 weeks-of-age (Dubbeldam, De Bakker and Bout 1995). Without their targets, the injured nerve fibers are unable to revert to a normal state, resulting in a possible heightened nociception by increased sensitization of nociceptors and form neuromas and generate spontaneous neural inputs in the amputated beak stump. Abnormal spontaneous activity has been found in the afferent fibers in the intramandibular nerve running from the stump to the trigeminal ganglia (Breward 1985; Breward and Gentle 1985). As found in rodents (Hu, Sessle, Raboisson, Dallel and Woda 1992), an expanding receptive field could been present in trigeminal brainstem neurons following beak-trimming. This abnormal plasticity in the neuronal system may lead to behavioral changes related to pain in trimmed birds, including exhibition of guarding behavior, i.e., reduction in environmental pecking, beak wiping, and head shaking when supplied drinking water at 45°C (Gentle, Thorp and Hughes 1995). Compared to the birds' behavior before beak-trimming and the behaviors of sham-operated controls, trimmed birds exhibited behavioral changes at least 5 weeks post trimming, almost certainly caused by pain (Duncan *et al.,* 1989). There were similar findings in cats and humans; lesion-induced sprouts in the distal stump of the nerve persisted for at least 18 months or for years

(Horch and Lisney 1981). However, Dubbeldam, Bout and De Bakker (1993) reported that there was no difference between controls and beak-trimmed birds in their tolerance to consume grain soaked with acetic acid that was used as a painful stimulus. Dubbeldam and Den Boer-Visser (1993) also reported that neuropeptide distribution, such as substance P and serotonin, which regulates pain sensation, in the primary sensory trigeminal nuclei did not differ between beak-trimmed birds and controls, suggesting that amputated beaks were not more susceptible to pain.

Factors that affect pain in beak-trimmed birds

Pain sensation varies among animals, which is affected by multiple factors such as the age of the bird when beak-trimming was performed, the type and size of lesions, the species or strains of birds, and individual characteristics (Table 3.3).

Beak-trimming pain *versus* phantom limb pain and stump pain

Phantom pain is painful sensations due to missing limb and other body parts, and stump pain is pain at the site of an extremity amputation. close to the scar (Browder and Gallagher 1948). As with amputation, beak-trimming, severs the distal portion of beak and causes damage to nerve fibers and beak tissue, which could result in pain that is similar to phantom limb pain and stump pain (Gentle 1986b; Gentle 1992).

Neuromas found in tissue stumps are a source of ectopic firing and trigger pain in human and rodent amputees. Similarly, neuromas with sensory corpuscles were found in the regrown beak stumps of brown egg hens beak-trimmed at 5 weeks-of-age or older (Gentle 1986a; Gentle, Waddington, Hunter and Jones 1990; Gentle, Hunter and Waddington 1991) and in White Leghorn x Australorp hens beak-trimmed at 1 day-of-age (Lunam, Glatz and Hsu 1996). Similar results have been obtained in male broiler-breeder chicks trimmed at hatch; the tip stump had a complete epidermal and dermal covering; the dermis was supplied with both nerve and blood vessels 22 days after beak-trimming (Gentle and Hunter 1988). Small neuromas also were found within the scar tissue of the stump and persisted over the 60-day observation period (Gentle and Hunter 1988). Abnormal afferent nerve fibers exhibiting spontaneous activity have also been found in the amputated beak stumps of Brown Leghorn birds beak-trimmed at 5 weeks-of-age (Breward

Table 3.3 Overview of some previous studies on the morphological and physiological changes of birds following beak-trimming

Breed/Strain	Age of beak-trimming	Amount of beak removed	Changes in nerve fibers	Neuroma formation and abnormal behaviors (pain)	References
Brown Leghorn	5 weeks	1/3 of upper and lower beak	spontaneous activity	developed by 15 days, well formed by 20-30 days post beak-trimming	Breward and Gentle, 1985
?	1 or 8 days, and 6 weeks	?	number of large fibers (↓) small myelinated fibers (↑) unmyelinated fiber (–)	heightened nociception	Dubbeldam et al. 1995
Brown Leghorn	16 weeks	? of both upper and lower beak		time spent feeding, drinking, and preening (↓); standing, inactive (↑); these changes last more than 5 weeks post beak-trimming	Duncan et al. 1989
Warren SSL Medium hybrids Brown Leghorn	80 weeks 40 weeks	1/3 to 1/2 of upper beak		decrease in food intake but no decline in feeding motivation	Gentle et al. 1982
Brown Leghorn	5 weeks	1/3 of upper and lower beak	nerve degeneration from 2-3 mm proximal to the stump; axon sprouts within 10 days	neuroma formed by 20-30 days post beak-trimming and become more extensive over the 70 day observation period	Gentle, 1986
Brown Leghorn	16 weeks	1/3 of upper and lower beak		during the "pain test", environmental pecking, beak wiping, and head shaking (↓); drinking (↓); hyperalgesia persisted for 6 weeks in beak-trimmed hens	Gentle et al. 1990

Table 3.3 Contd.

Breed/Strain	Age of beak-trimming	Amount of beak removed	Changes in nerve fibers	Neuroma formation and abnormal behaviors (pain)	References
Brown Leghorn	16 weeks	↑ of lower beak		massive injury discharge lasted from 2-48 sec; but no abnormal activity recorded from 90 to 270 min post beak-trimming	Gentle, 1991
Brown Leghorn	16 weeks	½ of upper and lower beak		reduction in the number of pecks at 26 h but not 6 h post beak-trimming	Gentle *et al.* 1991
Turkeys	1, 6, or 21 days	Bio-Beaker	devoid of afferent fibers and sensory nerve endings	no neuroma formation	Gentle *et al.* 1994
ISA Brown	1 or 10 days	1/3 of upper and lower beak	no scar tissue, no afferent nerves, no sensory corpuscles in beak stumps	no neuroma formation, less active, feed less, preened and less beak-related behaviors in trimmed birds	Gentle *et al.* 1997
Light strain (Steggles) and heavier strain (Hazlett)	30 weeks	3 mm of upper and lower beak		heart rate (↑) associated with beak-trimming related short term pain; food intake reduced for 9-10 days. Heavier strain took longer to recover than light strain from these effects of beak trimming.	Glatz, 1987
Crossbred chickens	6 weeks	1/3 of upper and lower beak		analgesics have the potential to maintain the feed intake of chickens in the first day after trimming, which may indicate that some of the acute pain had been relieved.	Glatz *et al.* 1992

Table 3.3 Contd.

Breed/Strain	Age of beak-trimming	Amount of beak removed	Changes in nerve fibers	Neuroma formation and abnormal behaviors (pain)	References
White Leghorn	4 weeks	¼ or ½ of upper and lower beak		more inactive and reduction in feeding behavior in chicken whose ½ beak was removed, respectively	Kuo and Craig, 1991
White Leghorn	4 weeks	½ of upper less lower beak		peck less at the feed, stood and crouched more in beak-trimmed chickens	Lee and Craig, 1990
White Leghorn × Australorp	1 day	Group 1. ½ of upper and 1/3 of lower		neuromas were present in the beaks of birds 10 weeks but not 70 weeks after beak-trimming; sensory corpuscles were present in both ages	Lunam et al. 1996
		Group 2. 2/3 of upper and ½ of lower beak		neuromas persisted in beaks of 70-week-old hens but sensory receptors were not seen in the beak stumps	

and Gentle 1985). The spontaneous firing is remarkably similar to the spontaneous discharges originating from stump neuromas in human amputees (Narsinghani and Anand 2000) and implicated in acute and chronic pain syndromes (Treede 1995; Wu and Chiu 1999). There are similar cellular mechanisms of neurogenic inflammation between birds and mammals, such as C-fiber nociceptors and pain conduction in the trigeminal nerves (Gentle and Hunter 1993; Eide and Rabben 1998; Bear, Connors and Paradiso 2001). In addition, similar trauma-induced morphological changes of trigeminal nerve fibers, i.e. a reduction in the density of large myelinated fibers and an increase in the number of small myelinated fibers, have been found in humans and birds (Dubbeldam *et al.,* 1995; Bear *et al.,* 2001). These changes may cause heightened nociception. The hypothesis is consistent with previous findings that Aδ-fibers are one of the small myelinated fibers and are involved in pain conduction by forming the most spontaneously active neuromas after amputation (Bear *et al.,* 2001). In neuromas, about 90% of all fibers are A-fibers (Holland and Robinson 1990; Coderre *et al.,* 1993). Based on these results, beak-trimming could result in pain exhibiting both acute and chronic patterns. Consistent with this hypothesis, Gentle *et al.* (1991) reported that a positive guarding behavior (protective behavior to avoid pain from tissue injury) was found in trimmed birds.

However, the hypothesis that beak-trimming-induced pathophysiological changes and pain are similar to those found in human amputees may need to be redefined. Post-amputation phenomena including painful and nonpainful phantom sensations occur following loss of limbs and other body parts, i.e., some devastating neuropathies are painless while other relatively small disorders are very painful (Wall 1981; Wall 1991; Weinstein 1998; Angrill and Koster 2000). The incidence of phantom limb pain ranges from less than 2% to nearly 100%, but severe phantom limb pain occurs in about only 5 to 10% of the cases (Weinstein 1998). Most phantom limb pain patients have a positive correlation with preamputation pain (Jensen, Krebs, Nielsen and Rasmussen 1983; Jensen, Krebs, Nielsen and Rasmussen 1984; Flor 2002; Frischenschlager and Pucher 2002). Preamputation pain results in long-term emotional memory of the painful experience (Angrill and Koster 2000). Lifelong phantom limb pain can be prevented through preemptive analgesia on patients with preamputation pain (Bloomquist 2001). On the other hand, prior to beak-trimming, a bird's beak is healthy and intact, and therefore the bird should have less or no sensation of pain. In addition, the development of phantom limb pain and stump pain depends on the type of myelinated afferent fibers involved. Tal, Wall and Devor (1999) reported that, in rats, spontaneous firing originating in neuromas was much more prevalent in the injured medial gastrocnemius nerve, a hindlimb muscle nerve, while there was no spontaneous discharge and very little ectopic mechanosensitivity in neuromas of the facial nerve, the motor branch of the trigeminal nerve that serves the striated muscles of the face. These differences may be related to the different spectrum of neuropathic symptomatology associated with nerve injury in the trigeminal fields vs. the segmental innervation fields (Tal *et al.,* 1999). A similar pain status, a relative silence in neuromas, may be present in beak-trimmed birds.

Beak-trimming in young *versus* old birds

Pain sensation and neuroma formation are affected by development of the nerve system which is age-dependent. Although neuromas and abnormal afferent fibers have been found in the beak stumps of birds trimmed at 5 weeks-of-age or older (Breward and Gentle 1985; Gentle 1986a; Gentle 1986b; Gentle *et al.,* 1990; Gentle *et al.,* 1991; Gentle 1992), it may not be the same in birds trimmed at an earlier age.

The major objection to beak-trimming is that it could induce formation of traumatic neuromas in beak stumps and that, in turn, could cause chronic pain, which is similar to phantom limb pain in humans. The hypothesis comes mostly from studies conducted by Gentle and his colleagues on Brown Egg layers whose beaks were trimmed at 5 weeks-of-age or older (Gentle 1989; Gentle *et al.,* 1990; Gentle *et al.,* 1991); their findings were reiterated by a study performed on younger chicks by the same authors (Gentle, Hughes, Fox and Waddington 1997) and in young turkeys (Gentle *et al.,* 1995). The authors reported that when chicks were beak-trimmed at either 1 or 10 days of age, unlike those trimmed at older ages, the beak healing process was faster with no scar tissue. The regrown tips did not contain afferent nerve or sensory corpuscles and there were no neuromas in the beak stumps at 3 and 6 wks after trimming. Desserich, Ziswiler and Folsch (1983; 1984; 1998), Blokhuis *et al.* (1998), Dubbeldam (1995) and Blokhuis and Wiepkema (1998) also reported that there were no neuromas in the beak stumps of birds trimmed at earlier ages. But there was an increase of small myelinated fibers in the beak stumps, which could indicate a high susceptibility to noxious stimuli (Dubbeldam *et al.,* 1995). However, Lunam, Glatz and Hsu (1996) reported that trauma-induced neuromas persisted in beaks of 10- and 70-week-old birds from the White Leghorn x Australorp strain after they were moderately or substantially trimmed at hatch, respectively (see Chapter 4 for beak-trimmed-induced changes in beak anatomy). Although these results reveal that neuroma formation and pain sensation are genetic (birds to be used)-and lesion (size of beak to be trimmed)-dependent, they may also be affected by differences in pain sensation, neural characteristics, and plasticity capability between young and old animals. These factors could lead to different reactions in response to beak-trimming among different age groups, which is similar to those found in humans and rodents, since the systems regulating stress response and pain thresholds are similar between birds and mammals (Eide and Rabben 1998; Bear *et al.*, 2001). In mammals, there are two major reasons, amongst others, for the differences in trauma-induced neuromas in different age groups: 1) in neonatal animals after amputation, most axotomized cells die in the dorsal root ganglia, while in adults, the majority of cells survive, and within a short time, axons sprout from retracted endbulbs from surviving cells to form neuromas; and 2) neuromas can regress and sometimes become microneuromas trapped within the stump, mostly an occurrence in young animals. These neuromas are difficult to see in routine nerve histology and are easily missed if special preparative techniques are not used, such as the application of specific neural tracers, such as biotinylated dextran amine, an anterograde neural tracer, and specific immunohistochemical stains, such as axon growth-associated protein-43. Axon growth-associated protein-43 has been used as a marker for axonal sprouting (Aigner and Caroni 1993; Benowitz and Routtenburg 1997; McNeill, Mori and Cheng 1999) and is found in neuromas following nerve damage (Schwob, Youngentob and Meiri 1994; Gilmer-Hill, Beuerman, Ma, Jiang, Tiel and Kline 2002).

Developmental morphological studies of the nervous system indicate that there are remarkable differences in neuronal plasticity in response to injury between neonates and adults. Previous hypothesis that neonates are unable to feel or to remember pain like that in adults has been reinforced (Abu-Saad, Bours, Stevens and Hamers 1998; Kostarczyk 1999; Puchalski and Nummel 2002). In mammals, such as humans and rodents, sensory nerve endings have been found in the skin of foetuses as early as 16 weeks (Fitzerald 1983; Anand and Hickey 1987), which indicates a potential presence of pain, even hyperalgesia, following nerve injury since the pain inhibitory descending system develops later or postnatally (Kostarczyk 1999; Narsinghani and Anand 2000). Adverse long-term effects of pain on the developing fetus and neonates have been identified, including permanent structural and function changes in the brain and spinal cord (Puchalski and Nummel 2002). Similar developments within the nerve system have been found in birds. The trigeminal ganglia, the site of the first order of sensory neurons that innervate the face and beak, develop when the embryo is two days old (Gaik and Farbman 1971a; Gaik and Farbman 1971b), and there was no differences in the types and number of trigeminal ganglial cells between birds 7 days post-hatch and adults. Using a horseradish peroxidase (HRP) analysis injection at axonal terminals, then analysis of HRP-filed neurons in the trigeminal ganglia), Noden (1980) showed that trigeminal nerve fibers fully develop prior to the third day post-hatch. These morphological studies revealed the possibility of inducing neuromas and pain even when beak-trimming is conduced at an earlier age. However, the duration of pain could be much shorter in young birds as compared to old birds. The cellular mechanisms underlying this state could be similar to those seen in humans and rodents. In humans, if neonates suffer tissue damage, they show fewer behavioral disturbances, and sensory function can be quickly restored without long-term chronic pain syndromes (Wall 1992). These differences in neonates are related to a later maturation of the nervous system and several other systems. In neonates, peripheral cutaneous innervation, neuroendocrine functions, and mechanisms that regulate inflammation still undergo developmental changes, which exhibit a great capability of plasticity in response to lesions. Based on these findings, beak-trimming currently is carried out either on newly hatched birds in the hatchery or when they are a few days old.

Pain *versus* the amount of beak removed

Previous studies have shown that sensation of pain and formation of neuromas in humans and other mammals depend on the type and/or severity of tissue injury (Bennett 1993; Sheen and Chung 1993; Colburn, Rickman and DeLeo 1999). In birds, as in mammals, the persistence of neuromas depends on the severity of tissue damage, such as the amount of beak removed during trimming. Lunam *et al.* (1996) reported that following a moderate beak-trimming (half of the upper beak and one-third of the lower beak) in the White Leghorn x Australorp birds at hatch caused trauma-induced neuromas in the beaks of birds 10-weeks-old but not 70-weeks-old, and the distribution of nerves around the blood vessels and in the dermis were normal. Following a severe beak-trimming (two-thirds of the upper beak and half of the lower beak) at hatch, trauma-induced neuromas persisted in 70-week-old birds (Lunam *et al.,* 1996). Similarly, Gentle, Hughes, Fox and Waddington (1997) reported the absence of gross and microscopic morphopathological changes in beaks subjected to a mild trim, i.e., no neuromas and scar tissue, and regrowth with anatomically normal dermis with various sensory receptors, Herbst and Grandry corpuscles, and free nerve endings in the beak stumps. These beak stump characteristics suggest that less chronic pain is present in birds after a moderate beak-trimming. Based on these previous studies, it is currently recommended that only one-third to half of the beak should be trimmed.

Conclusion

Beak-trimming may cause pain (acute, chronic, or both) in trimmed birds due to tissue damage and nerve injury. The complexity and plasticity of the nervous system and the animal's inability to communicate verbally make pain difficult to measure directly. However, pain in animals can be recognized and assessed using physiological and behavioral parameters in response to noxious events. When evaluating whether an animal is experiencing pain, it should be noted that beak-trimming-induced pain in birds is genetic-, lesion-, and age-dependent.

4

The anatomy and innervation of the chicken beak: effects of trimming and re-trimming

Christine A. Lunam

Summary

This chapter reviews the microanatomy of the beak of the domestic chicken and the anatomical consequences of the practice of beak-trimming. The chicken beak is a complex organ which is extensively innervated by sensory, sympathetic and parasympathetic nerves. The salivary glands and their associated taste buds receive parasympathetic and sensory innervation respectively whilst the rich vascular network is innervated by sympathetic and parasympathetic nerves. Free nerve endings serve as nociceptors that respond to noxious stimuli. The sensory receptors, the Herbst and Grandry corpuscles, are concentrated in the region of the beak tip and are innervated by branches from the trigeminal nerve.

Beak-trimming removes the majority of the sensory receptors and severs the innervating axons. The regenerating nerves in the beak stump develop traumatic neuromas that consist of an entwining mass of regenerating axon sprouts. They may persist either as large masses or form scattered multiple fascicles of axons. The severed axons regrow, the excess axon sprouts degenerate and the neuroma regresses. However, a critical amount of beak tissue can be removed beyond which neuromas will not resolve. Moderate trimming and re-trimming results in resorption of scar tissue and allows sufficient peripheral targets to accommodate the regenerating axon sprouts. The regenerated tissue is re-innervated and free nerve endings as well as sensory receptors are present at the beak tip.

Introduction

The avian beak is a complex structure that undertakes a wide range of tasks pivotal to the normal physiological and social behaviour of birds. The beak is not only essential for eating and drinking, but serves to grasp and discriminate between food particles. It is also used for grooming, nesting and for aggressive and defensive activities. To accommodate this diverse range of tasks the beak contains a variety of anatomical features. These include specialised sensory receptors, nerves, blood vessels, salivary glands and associated taste buds. A detailed description of the gross anatomy and histology of beaks of different bird species is provided by Lucas and Stettenheim (1972). This chapter will focus on the microanatomy of the beak of the domestic chicken and the anatomical consequences of the practice of beak-trimming which involves partial removal of the upper and lower beak. For a detailed discussion of the effects of beak-trimming on behaviour see Chapter 5 of this volume.

Microanatomy of the beak

Both the upper and lower beak of the chicken form a sharp tip with the upper beak forming a curved extension over the lower beak. Structural support of the upper beak is provided by the premaxillary bone, which extends to the beak tip. The lower beak is supported by fusion of the mandibular bones. The external surface of the chicken beak is covered by the rhamphotheca, an acellular keratinised layer that in the upper beak is particularly thickened at the tip. The keratin of both the upper and lower beak extends over the sharp tomial edges. Immediately beneath the rhamphotheca lies the epidermis that consists of several layers of epithelial cells. The basal cells of the epidermis undergo cell division, and as they migrate towards the surface they become flattened, produce keratohyalin granules and finally degenerate to form the rhamphotheca.

Between the epidermis and the collagenous periosteum of the bone lies the dermis. It consists of dense collagen and elastic fibres in which are embedded numerous arteries and veins, nerve fibres and sensory receptors. Dermal papillae penetrate into the epidermis at the beak tip and in the lower beak extend into the rhamphotheca. A feature of the dorsal surface of the upper beak is the presence of dermal papillae invested by numerous capillaries that project deeply into the epidermis. The microanatomy of the upper beak is shown in Figure 4.1A-C.

Innervation

The upper and lower beak receives sensory, sympathetic and parasympathetic innervation. A detailed account of the innervation of the chicken beak is given by King and McLelland (1975) and Akester (1979). The upper beak

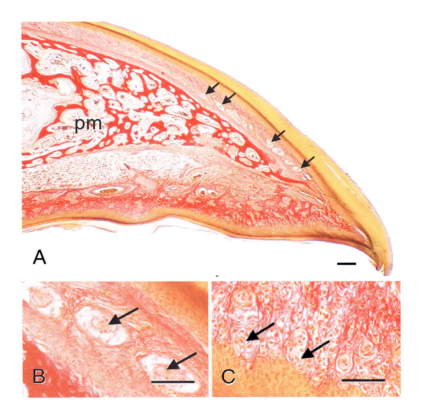

Figure 4.1A-C Sagittal sections through the upper beak of a day-old chicken stained with Verhoeff and van Gieson. **(A)** Shows the rhamphotheca covering of the dorsal surface. Note the increasing thickness of the rhamphotheca as it approaches the beak tip. Large Herbst corpuscles (arrows) lie in the dense collagenous connective tissue between the premaxillary bone (pm) and the epidermis. **(B)** Herbst corpuscles within the dorsal dermis have a dense inner core (arrows) surrounded by pale staining lamellae. **(C)** Grandry corpuscles (arrows) lie within the dermal papillae adjacent to the epidermis (e) lining the upper palate. The Grandry corpuscles are comprised of stacks of Grandry cells orientated perpendicular to the long axis of the beak. Scale bar = 200µm for Figure 4.1A. Scale bars = 100µm for Figures 4.1B and 4.1C.

receives sensory afferents via the ophthalmic branch of the trigeminal nerve (Figure 4.4A). It also receives parasympathetic and sensory innervation from the facial nerve. Sensory afferents of the facial nerve are from the geniculate ganglion whereas the parasympathetic innervation is via the dorsal sphenopalatine and ethmoid ganglia. The lower beak also receives dual sensory innervation via the intramandibular branch of the trigeminal nerve and from the chorda tympani branch of the facial nerve (Gentle 1984). The anterior region of the lower beak is innervated by parasympathetic fibres from the mandibular ganglion. Sympathetic innervation to the vascular smooth muscle in the mucosa of the upper and lower beak is via the cranial cervical ganglion.

Salivary glands

Secretion of salivary mucus is particularly important to grain feeding birds. The chicken has extensive salivary acini in the anterior regions of the upper and lower beaks and in the tongue (Nickel, Schummer and Seiferle 1977). The maxillary (Figure 4.2A-C), palatine and sphenopterygoid glands are located in the upper beak, the anterior (rostral) and posterior mandibular glands are situated in the lower beak with the anguli oris glands at the angle of the mouth. Lingual salivary glands are present in the tongue.

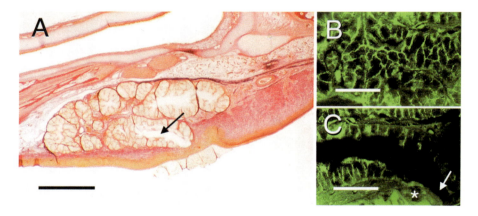

Figure 4.2A-C Sagittal sections through the maxillary salivary gland within the upper beak of a day-old chicken. (A) The section shown has been stained with Verhoeff and van Gieson and reveals extensive pale mucous acini. The salivary duct (arrow) projects distally towards the palate. Salivary mucus is visible on the surface of the palate in the region of the opening of the duct. (B) Nerve fibres showing immunoreactivity for substance P (SP), visible by green fluorescence, are numerous both amongst the salivary acini and (C) lining the salivary duct. SP-IR nerve fibres are absent within the taste bud (asterisk) located in the epithelium adjacent to the duct opening (arrow). Sections were incubated in rabbit antiserum raised against SP followed by incubation with sheep anti-rabbit IgG conjugated to fluorescein isothiocyanate. Scale bar = 2mm for Figure 4.2A. Scale bars = 500 µm for Figures 4.2B and 4.2C.

In contrast to mammals, the saliva in the chicken consists solely of mucus, devoid of amylase (Jerrett and Goodge 1973) and takes little part if any, in initial digestion. In addition to providing protection from micro-organisms the saliva coats the ingested feed particles that are then thrown onto the palate to form a bolus prior to being swallowed (Gargiulo, Lorvik, Ceccarelli and Pedini 1991). Parasympathetic innervation and control of salivary gland secretion is considered to be by branches of the facial and glossopharyngeal nerves (Bolton 1976). Parasympathetic innervation of the salivary glands of the upper beak is considered to be from the ethmoid and sphenopalatine ganglia (Akester 1979) whereas parasympathetic secretomotor fibres via the mandibular ganglion within the chorda tympani nerve innervate the salivary glands of lower beak (King and McLelland, 1975; Bubien-Waluszewska 1981).

Taste buds

Domestic fowl are fastidious feeders. Vision, texture of the feed and taste are all important cues used in feed selection by fowl (Kare and Rogers 1976; Gentle 1979). In chickens taste buds are most numerous in the palate and in the anterior mandibular region (Ganchrow and Ganchrow 1986; Saito 1966). They have a similar structure to other vertebrates and lie in close proximity to the salivary ducts (Gentle 1971; Lindenmaier and Kare 1959; Saito 1966; Lunam and Glatz 1995a; Lunam and Glatz 1993).

Taste buds in the chicken, similar to mammalian taste buds, rely on extrinsic sensory innervation to maintain their structural and functional integrity (Gentle 1971; Ganchrow and Ganchrow, 1986). In the upper beak they receive sensory innervation by the greater superficial petrosal nerve and in the anterior mandibular region of the lower beak by the chorda tympani branch of the facial nerve (Ganchrow, Gentle and Ganchrow 1987; Gentle 1983).

Gentle (1971) using silver staining techniques observed nerve fibres branching from a plexus at the base of the bud that penetrate into lingual taste buds of the chicken. A double-labelling immunohistochemical study (Lunam and Glatz 1993) examined the distribution of the neuropeptide substance P (SP) and calbindin, a calcium binding protein, in the upper chicken beak. The taste buds in the upper beak had a similar structure to the lingual taste buds in the chicken reported by Gentle (1971). Lunam and Glatz (1993) identified intragemmal nerve fibres labelling for calbindin in the taste buds adjacent to the opening of salivary ducts in the maxillary gland. Calbindin immmunoreactive nerve fibres were also present in the salivary duct and in the dermis amongst the salivary acini. Whereas the salivary gland was invested by a dense plexus of periacinar nerve fibres immunoreactive for SP, in contrast to mammalian taste buds (Yamamoto, Nagai, Shimura and Yasoshima 1998), no nerve fibres labelling for SP were observed within the buds (Figure 4.2B-C). This study demonstrates that although the structure and physiology of avian taste buds is similar to those of mammals, differences in the neurochemical content of the innervating sensory afferents exist between the two vertebrate classes.

Lunam and Glatz (1993) reported the presence of intra-acinar ganglia within the chicken maxillary gland that contained two distinct neurochemical populations. They proposed that the intra-acinar cell bodies (presumably post-ganglionic parasympathetic neurons) have dual projections; SP-containing neurons innervate the salivary acini whereas calbindin-labelled neurons project to the taste buds. This raises the possibility in the chicken that in addition to extrinsic innervation, a local neuronal circuit exists between the salivary acini and taste buds.

Encapsulated sensory receptors

The beak of Aves contains two types of encapsulated sensory receptors, the Herbst and Grandry corpuscles (Figures 4.1A-C and 4.4A; see review by Gottschaldt 1985). Herbst corpuscles have a structure and physiology similar to mammalian Pacinian corpuscles. They are ovoid and are comprised of a lamella of circularly arranged collagen fibres with an inner core of specialised Schwann cells. After entering the collagen capsule the myelinated afferent nerve weaves into the core of the corpuscle where it finally loses its myelin sheath. Grandry corpuscles consist of an enclosed stack of specialised cells (Grandry cells) innervated by a series of terminals from a myelinated sensory afferent nerve. Grandry cells within the corpuscle are histologically similar to mammalian intraepidermal Merkel cells. This has led to confusion in the terminology Grandry and Merkel corpuscles. The term Grandry corpuscles was proposed for all avian sensory corpuscles containing morphologically distinguishable Grandry cells (Ide and Munger 1978).

Ultrastructural studies have revealed the fine structural detail of these mechanoreceptors in the avian beak (Andersen and Nafstad 1968; Nafstad 1971; Saxod 1978). Both the Herbst and Grandry corpuscles are rapidly adapting mechanoreceptors found predominantly in the beak and in feathered skin of Aves (reviewed by Gottschaldt 1985). In the beak they are innervated by large diameter sensory afferents from the trigeminal nerve.

Herbst and Grandry corpuscles in the beak of the pigeon and of the duck are innervated by nerves labelling for calcium binding proteins (Del Valle, Ciriaco, Bronzetti, Albuerne, Naves, Germana and Vega 1995). A recent ultrastructural immunohistochemical study reported the distribution of calcium binding proteins in the axons innervating Herbst and Grandy corpuscles in the beak skin of the duck (Chouchkov, Palov and Dandov 2002). It is generally accepted that calcium binding proteins may participate in transduction mechanisms of the sensory mechanoreceptors by regulating levels of intracellular free calcium. Similar to the presence of calcium binding proteins in the sensory afferents innervating the encapsulated corpuscles in the beak of pigeons and the duck bill, work in our laboratory has demonstrated calbindin in the sensory afferents innervating Herbst and Grandry corpuscles in the chicken beak (unpublished data). Gentle (1989) revealed that Herbst and Grandry corpuscles in the chicken beak have similar electrophysiological properties to those of other avian species. It is considered that these sensory receptors respond to mechanical stimuli and also provide fine tactile discrimination, allowing selection of food and non-food particles.

Distribution of receptors

In the upper beak of the chicken (Gentle, Hughes, Fox and Waddington 1997) and the turkey (Gentle, Thorp and Hughes 1995), Herbst and Grandry corpuscles have a similar somatotopic distribution. Both receptors decrease in number from the tip to the nares (Figure 4.2A-C). The Herbst corpuscles lie in the dermis dorsal to the perichondrium of the premaxillary bone. These tend to be the largest corpuscles, measuring 120-200 µm in diameter in the chicken. Large Herbst corpuscles are also found in the dorsal surface close to the beak tip. Many smaller Herbst corpuscles, 20-80 µm in diameter, reside in the dermis ventral to the premaxillary bone (adjacent to the roof of the oral cavity) and near the beak tip. Grandry corpuscles are numerous in the ventral dermis and tend to lie within dermal papillae and in the dermis at the beak tip.

In the lower beak of the chicken, large Herbst corpuscles lie in the dorsal dermis near the beak tip and rapidly decrease in number with an occasional Herbst corpuscle located near the anterior mandibular salivary glands. Grandry corpuscles lie in the dermis adjacent to the floor of the oral cavity. Both Herbst and Grandry corpuscles are concentrated in the bill tip organ.

Bill tip organ

At the tip of the lower beak dermal papillae are arranged into parallel arrays that extend into the rhamphotheca to form the bill tip organ. The bill tip organ has been described in a variety of avian species including the goose (Gottschaldt and Lausmann 1974) and the duck (Berkhoudt 1976; Berkhoudt 1980). In contrast to the goose and duck, where the bill tip organ is present in both the upper and lower beak, in the chicken it is present only in the lower beak. A detailed account of the bill tip organ in the chicken is given by Gentle and Breward (1986). The papillae contain nerves, blood vessels and sensory receptors. Grandry corpuscles are concentrated in the distal region of the papillae whilst Herbst corpuscles are most numerous proximally. The specialised dermal papillae are thought to enhance tactile discrimination (Gottschaldt and Lausmann 1974; Gentle and Breward 1986).

Free nerve endings

In addition to the encapsulated sensory mechanoreceptors, the beak also contains free nerve endings. These are the terminals of unmyelinated C-fibres and small diameter myelinated A-delta sensory afferents of the trigeminal nerve. Free nerve endings in the chicken beak are located in the dermis near the dermal-epidermal border and are numerous in the tip of the upper beak (Andersen and Nafstad 1968; Lunam, Glatz and Hsu 1996; Gentle *et al.*, 1997) and in the bill tip organ of the lower beak (Gentle and Breward 1986). Immunohistochemical studies have provided evidence of different populations of free nerve endings in the chicken beak that can be distinguished by their different neuropeptide content. Lunam and Glatz (1995b) reported individual nerve fibres labelled for either SP or calcitonin gene-related peptide (CGRP) whereas both neuropeptides co-existed in other free nerve endings.

SP and CGRP are found in mammalian primary afferent nerves and physiological studies have provided evidence that they serve as peptidergic neurotransmitters in nociceptive responses (Lu, Park, Rice and Laurito 2003). Furthermore, in mammals the differential release of SP and CGRP to thermal, electrical and to noxious stimuli demonstrate that these peptides predominantly serve unmyelinated C-fibre nociceptors (Lawson 1995). In view of the correlation between neuropeptide content and physiological characteristics observed in mammalian nociceptors, the presence of free nerve endings labelling for SP and CGRP in the chicken beak suggest that they serve as avian nociceptors.

In support of this notion, Gentle and Hunter (1993) demonstrated intraepidermal injection of SP, external application of mustard oil or thermal and mechanical stimuli to the wattle, as well as antidromic stimulation of trigeminal C-fibre nociceptors, produces plasma extravasation, a feature of the mammalian inflammatory response. Similar responses are observed with neurogenic inflammation in mammals following electrical, mechanical and noxious stimuli of C-fibre nociceptors (Greenspan 1997; Sann, Harti, Pierau and Simon 1987; Sann and Pierau 1998). Earlier electrophysiological studies (Breward 1983) demonstrated the presence of thermal nociceptors and sensory receptors that respond to thermal and noxious stimuli, in the chicken beak. Gentle (1989, 1991) further characterised nociceptors in the chicken beak, with similar response characteristics to those found in mammals, into mechano-thermal (C fibre) and high threshold mechanical nociceptors (both C and A-delta fibres).

Capsaicin is extracted from hot chilli peppers. In mammals, capsaicin sensitises and activates C and A-delta nociceptors inducing the release of SP from sensory afferent nerves. It binds to the vanilloid/capsaicin receptor which is selectively expressed in mammalian primary afferent nociceptors (for review see Basbaum, Julius and Robbins, 2003). In contrast, capsaicin induces mild behavioural responses in birds (Mason and Maruniak 1983). Indeed, Avian species demonstrate a preference for capsaicin. Red-winged blackbirds preferentially select drinking water containing capsaicin (Mason and Maruniak, 1983) and chickens exhibit a preference for feed mixed with capsaicin (Lunam and Glatz 1995a). In the pigeon, capsaicin did not result in release of SP from either the spinal cord (Szolcsanyi, Sann and Pierau 1986) or from sensory afferents (Pierau, Gamse, Harti and Gamse 1987). Gentle and Hunter (1993) argued that the insensitivity of birds to the noxious effects of capsaicin is likely due to the lack of a capsaicin receptor rather than to a difference in the physiological response of the sensory fibres. In support of Gentle and Hunter's argument, a difference in the domain that confers sensitivity to capsaicin has been identified between the vanilloid receptors of Aves and mammals (Jordt and Julius 2002). Furthermore, the release of SP from mammalian nociceptors occurs with acute inflammation (Sann and Pierau 1998) and recent immunohistochemical evidence suggests that SP is released in response to acute inflammation from sensory nerve endings in the chicken (Lunam and Gentle 2004). This study provides further support that Avian and mammalian nociceptors have similar physiological responses.

The existence of sensory trigeminal afferent fibres with similar electrophysiological properties characteristic of mammalian peripheral nociceptors and the presence of free nerve endings labelling for SP and CGRP in the chicken beak suggest these peptides are neurotransmitters in polymodal nociceptors.

Summary

In summary, the chicken beak is a highly specialised organ containing salivary glands and taste buds to assist feeding and taste discrimination as well as thermoreceptors, mechanoreceptors and nociceptors that respond to thermal, mechanical and noxious stimuli. The encapsulated mechanoreceptors, the Herbst and Grandry corpuscles, are concentrated near the tip of the upper beak and in the lower beak are incorporated into the bill tip organ, a sensory structure that is considered to enhance fine tactile discrimination. The beak is well innervated by sensory, parasympathetic and sympathetic nerves and contains numerous free nerve endings within the dermis of the tip of the upper beak and bill tip organ

Effect of beak-trimming

Beak-trimming involves partial removal of the upper and lower beak usually with an electrically-heated blade. The anatomical consequences of beak-trimming have been investigated in the chicken (Gentle 1986; Lunam and Glatz 1995a, 1997; Lunam *et al.,* 1996; Gentle *et al.,* 1997) and the turkey (Gentle and Hughes 1995; Gentle 1986b). Trimming results in severing of blood vessels and nerves, removal of bone, dermis, epidermis and rhamphotheca. Excessive trimming would result also in removal of the salivary glands. Fibroelastic scar tissue mixed with congealed blood forms over the wound. Within several days after trimming, the epidermis regenerates and commences to grow over the scar tissue, which will eventually be replaced by the regenerating dermis (Gentle 1986a; Lunam *et al.,* 1996; Gentle *et al.,* 1997). The ability of the beak to regrow is dependent on the species of bird, the age of the bird at the time of trimming, the amount of tissue removed and the extent of damage proximal to the site of cutting caused by cautery.

To assess the effects of beak-trimming on the well-being of the bird, numerous studies have investigated its effects on behaviour, physiology and the microanatomy of the beak. For a recent overview of beak-trimming in chickens see Jendral and Robinson (2004).

Two major welfare issues arise from beak-trimming. The first is loss of sensory input to the beak as a consequence of removal of sensory receptors. The second issue is the potential for acute and chronic pain as a result of severing nerves within the beak. The following discussion will address the microanatomy of the beak after trimming and re-trimming with a focus on removal of the sensory receptors and nerve regeneration. In particular, the influence of age of trimming and the amount of tissue removed on the microanatomy of the beak will be reviewed. The potential welfare implications of the histopathology of the beak are addressed.

Encapsulated sensory receptors

A consequence of beak-trimming is the removal of sensory receptors that are concentrated at the beak tip in the chicken and the turkey. Discrepancies exist in the literature as to whether sensory receptors regrow within the beak tip after trimming. Several studies have reported permanent removal of sensory receptors after beak-trimming (Cunningham 1992; Gentle 1986a; Gentle 1986b) with a loss of sensory input. The loss of sensory input has been correlated with a reduction in feed intake (Glatz and Lunam 1994) and pecking efficiency (Gentle, Hughes and Hubrecht 1982). In addition, the absence of sensory receptors at the beak tip is associated with a permanent significant loss of temperature and touch responses (Gentle 1986a) thereby having a detrimental affect on the long-term welfare of the bird.

Studies indicate that the age at which beak-trimming is conducted and the amount of tissue removed significantly influences the presence of sensory receptors in the regrown beaks.

Gentle (1986b) examined the histology of the beaks of Brown Leghorn birds trimmed at five weeks-of-age. In this study one-third of the upper and lower beaks were removed. Following trimming, the dermis was devoid of sensory receptors and free nerve endings. The beaks consisted entirely of scar tissue that persisted to 70 days-of-age.

In contrast, trimming at a younger age results in rapid regeneration of the beak tissue with minimal formation of scar tissue. In an anatomical and behavioural study Gentle *et al.* (1997) investigated the effects of removal of one-third of the upper and lower beaks of ISA Brown chicks at either one or 10 days-of-age. Forty–two days after trimming the upper beaks were found to be devoid of scar tissue. Although nerves and sensory corpuscles were observed within the dermis of the regenerated tissue, these were absent at the beak tip. Despite differences in beak length after regrowth, all beak-trimmed birds demonstrated similar reductions in feather pecking. Gentle and colleagues therefore argued that the observed reduction in feather pecking after trimming resulted from sensory deprivation at the beak tip rather than by a decrease in beak length. These conclusions are supported by Hughes and Michie (1982) who reported the reduction in feather pecking after trimming was unrelated to differences in the beak length.

The enhanced ability of the chicken beak to regenerate after trimming at an early age, and the absence of receptors and afferent nerve fibres at the tip of the beak following regrowth has also been observed in the turkey. Removal of one–third of the upper beak of turkeys at either one, six or 21 days-of-age resulted in extensive beak regrowth with minimal scar tissue 42 days after trimming (Gentle *et al.,* 1995; Gentle and Hughes 1995).

Permanent loss of sensory receptors and the absence of free nerve endings in the beak tip after trimming at an early age is not consistently observed. In Tegel Tint hens moderately trimmed (half of the upper and one-third of the lower beak) on the day of hatch, free nerve endings and sensory receptors have been observed in the beak tip (Lunam and Glatz 1995a; Lunam and Glatz 1997; Lunam *et al.,* 1996). Herbst and Grandry corpuscles as well as free nerve endings, although fewer in number compared to those in the non-trimmed beaks, were observed at 10 and 70 weeks after trimming. In comparison, beaks severely trimmed on the day of hatch had extensive scar tissue and receptors were absent in the regrown stumps (Figure 4.4B).

Re-trimming

Re-trimming is an industry practice conducted to decrease cannibalistic feather pecking following beak regrowth. An anatomical and behavioural study examined the effects of moderate beak-trimming of chickens on the day of hatch and re-trimming of 2mm at 14 weeks-of-age (Lunam, Glatz and Barnett 1998). Sensory receptors and individual nerve fibres were observed near the tips of the trimmed upper and lower beaks at 28 weeks-of-age. In the tip of the lower beak, large Herbst corpuscles were present and many nerve bundles traversed the dermis between the mandibular bone and epidermis of the beak tip (Figure 4.3A-B).

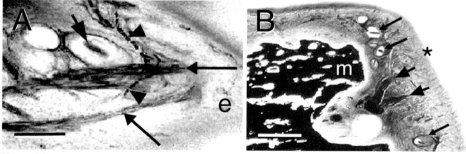

Figure 4.3A-B Silver impregnation of sagittal sections showing the region of the tip of the lower beak from hens at 28 weeks-of-age. **(A)** One-third of the beak was trimmed at hatch. Nerve fibres (arrows) are present in the dermis and extend to the epidermis (e). The innervating nerve fibre (short arrow) within the central core of a large Herbst corpuscle is visible. Arrowheads indicate a capillary within the dermis. **(B)** Re-trimmed (2mm) at 14 weeks-of-age. The beak is considerably blunter compared to the thin taper observed after a single trimming. The mandibular bone (m) lies within 500μm of the epidermis (asterisk) at the beak tip. Numerous Herbst corpuscles (long arrows) lie in the dermis between the bone and beak tip. The innervating nerve of each corpuscle is shown as a central dark band. Nerve bundles (short arrows) traverse the dermis adjacent to the Herbst corpuscles. Scale bar = 100μm for Figure 4.3A. Scale bar = 500μm for Figure 4.3B.

At 66 weeks-of-age, sensory receptors and nerve fibres were observed in the dermis at the beak tip (Glatz, Lunam, Barnett and Jongman 1998). That the hens returned to normal feeding and pecking behaviours by 66 weeks-of-age supports the microanatomy as it suggests that sensory input to the beak is at least partially restored.

Taken collectively the data suggest that moderate trimming at hatch or at an early age, as well as conservative re-trimming at 14 weeks-of-age minimises the development of scar tissue and allows reinnervation of free nerve endings into the beak tip. In addition, some of the encapsulated sensory receptors in the beak stump will gradually move towards the beak tip with regeneration of the dermis. In some cases, the receptors will reach the tip of the beak.

Innervation

Acute and chronic pain after beak-trimming is a significant welfare issue and as such has been the focus of numerous anatomical, electrophysiological and behavioural studies. Evaluation of the effect of beak-trimming is confounded as pain resulting from peripheral nerve injury is a complex phenomenon that evokes events in the peripheral and central nervous systems (reviewed by Cervero and Laird 2003; Colburn and Munglani 2003). It is well established that the sensation of pain ultimately arises from interpretation within the brain of signals arriving from the periphery. In mammals a wealth of evidence exists demonstrating peripheral nerve injury may result in reorganisation of neural connections in the spinal cord, excitation of peripheral nerves distant from the site of injury, as well as the formation of new connections to the central neural tracts.

In birds, anatomical studies have dealt only with the peripheral effects of beak-trimming. Therefore the histopathology observed after beak-trimming does not provide conclusive evidence that birds experience pain. To assess the welfare consequences of beak-trimming the histopathology needs to be correlated with electrophysiological and behavioural data (discussed elsewhere in this volume, in Chapters 3 and 5). The following discussion focuses on the anatomical effects of trimming on the sensory nerves within the beak.

Nociceptors

It is well established that the tip of the beak contains many free nerve endings with neuropeptides and electrophysiological properties characteristic of nociceptors. Beak-trimming severs the axons of the free nerve endings. Electrophysiological studies have demonstrated excitation of nociceptors at the time of beak-trimming (Breward, 1983) followed by a period of several hours devoid of abnormal neural discharges (Gentle, 1991). Similar responses, associated with acute pain, are observed in humans after nerve damage. In addition, sensitisation of nociceptors after nerve injury is considered to evoke hyperalgesia (decreased threshold to stimuli) and allodynia, a perception where normally non-noxious stimuli become painful. In birds, behavioural evidence consistent with acute and persistent pain (hyperalgesia and guarding behaviour) is observed after beak-trimming (Gentle, Waddington, Hunter and Jones 1990; Duncan, Slee, Seawright and Breward 1989). On balance, anatomical, electrophysiological and behavioural evidence strongly suggest that beak-trimming evokes acute pain.

Neuromas

A major welfare concern is the development of traumatic neuromas by the regenerating fibres in the beak stump (Figures 4.4B, 4.5A-B). These have been implicated as a cause of chronic pain after beak-trimming in the chicken (Breward and Gentle 1985; Gentle 1986a; Lunam *et al.,* 1996). The basis for this, is that neuromas generate spontaneous neural activity in hens (Breward and Gentle 1985) and similar discharges result in chronic neuroma pain in mammals (Devor and Rappaport 1990).

In mammals, traumatic neuromas develop after severing of peripheral axons. The development, histology and pathophysiology of neuromas are reviewed by Devor and Rappaport (1990). Briefly, this involves initial degeneration, then sprouting of the regenerating axons to form disorganised tangles of nerves. The regenerating axon sprouts may form as either large masses (Figures 4.4B and 4.5B) or may develop as small scattered multiple fascicles of axons to form microneuromas (Figure 4.5A). After several weeks, the nerve fibres regrow, the excess axon sprouts degenerate and the neuroma regresses. Neuromas may persist and discharge ectopic spontaneous action potentials that are perceived as chronic pain.

Risk factors

In Aves as in mammals, the extent to which neuromas develop and the length of time they persist, depends on the age at which the injury occurred, the

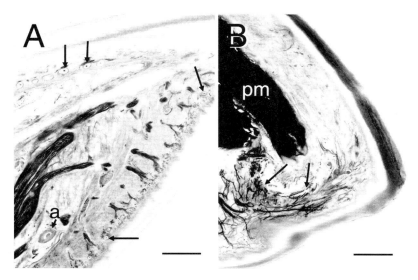

Figure 4.4A-B Silver impregnation of sagittal sections from the upper beak. **(A)** Non-trimmed beak at 28 weeks-of-age. Nerve fibres (stained black) run in parallel arrays. Large nerve bundles lie in the centre of the section with smaller bundles branching to innervate structures in the ventral dermis adjacent to the roof of the palate. Small and large Herbst corpuscles are shown in the ventral and dorsal surfaces respectively (arrows). A large artery (a) lies beneath the centrally located nerve bundles. **(B)** This section shows an extensive neuroma (arrows) in the beak of an adult hen severely trimmed on the day of hatch. The neuroma consists of a mass of disorganised nerve fibres ventral to the premaxillary bone (pm). Sensory receptors are absent. Scale bars = 500μm for Figures 4.4A and 4.4B.

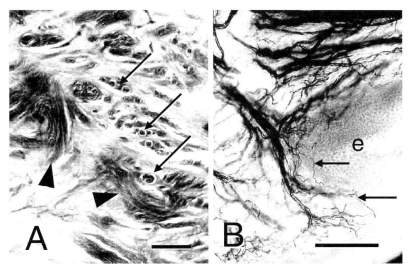

Figure 4.5A-B Silver impregnation of sections of the upper beak of adult hens showing neuromas after beak-trimming at hatch. **(A)** Microneuromas are visible as multiple clusters of small nerve bundles orientated sagittally (arrowheads) and transversely (arrows) to the plane of sectioning. **(B)** This micrograph shows numerous disorganised nerve fibres formed by sprouting of severed axons from a persistent traumatic neuromal mass after severe trimming. Individual axons (arrows) penetrate the epidermis (e). Scale bars = 100μm for Figures 4.5A and 4.5B.

amount of scar tissue formed, which effectively blocks the path of the regenerating sprouts, and the removal of the peripheral targets of the developing axon sprouts (Lunam and Glatz 1997; Lunam *et al.,* 1996). An individual susceptibility exists in many species to the length of time it may take for the neuroma to resolve. The neuroma may persist for many months or even years after nerve damage. Such variability in the time taken for the neuroma to resolve is well documented in humans after nerve injury (Flor, Devor and Jensen 2003), in emu toes after declawing (Lunam and Glatz 2000) and in beaks of domestic fowl after trimming (Lunam *et al.,* 1996).

Age of trimming

An absence of neuromas and scar tissue has been reported in the beaks of adult chickens (White Leghorn x Australorp) after trimming of one-half of the upper beak and one-third of the lower beak on the day of hatch (Lunam *et al.,* 1996). Similarly beaks of ISA Brown chickens trimmed at either one or 10 days-of-age (Gentle *et al.,* 1997) or turkeys trimmed at one, six or 21 days-of-age (Gentle *et al.,* 1995) showed no evidence of either neuromas or scar formation 42 days after trimming. In these studies by Gentle and colleagues (1995, 1997) one-third of the upper and lower beaks were removed.

In contrast to the above studies, neuromas have been reported in beaks of birds trimmed at an older age. Gentle (1986b) reported neuromas and extensive scar tissue in the upper beak of Brown Leghorn hens following removal of one-third of the beak at 5 weeks-of-age. Neuromas were present three weeks after trimming and had become more extensive by 10 weeks after trimming. As the beaks were not examined beyond 10 weeks after trimming, it is not known whether the neuromas would have eventually resolved.

The evidence above suggests that beak-trimming at a young age decreases the formation of scar tissue and reduces the risk of neuroma development. A likely explanation for this phenomenon is that the beak of young birds has a greater capacity for regeneration compared to the regenerative ability of older birds.

Severity of trimming

Evidence indicates that in addition to age of trimming, the amount of tissue removed has a significant influence on the development of neuromas and their subsequent potential for resolution.

Studies suggest that conservative trimming minimises the risk of neuroma development. Neither neuromas nor scar tissue was observed six weeks after trimming one-third of the upper and lower beaks of either day-old chickens (Gentle *et al.,* 1997) or turkeys (Gentle *et al.,* 1995).

In contrast, we observed microneuromas in beaks of chickens at 10 weeks-of-age that had been moderately trimmed (removal of one-half of the upper beak and one-third of the lower beak) on the day of hatch (Lunam *et al.,* 1996). These reported discrepancies in neuroma development are unlikely to result from either strain or species differences, as neuromas were not observed in trimmed beaks of different strains of domestic fowl or in the turkey. A more plausible explanation is that the initial development of neuromas depends on the amount of tissue removed. In our studies one-half of the upper beak was removed compared to one-third by other workers.

Furthermore, by 70 weeks-of-age, neuromas were not observed after moderate trimming at hatch, whereas neuromas and extensive scar tissue were present in beaks that had been severely trimmed (removal of two-thirds of the upper beak and one-half lower beak; Figures 4.4B and 4.5B) on the day of hatch (Lunam *et al.,* 1996). As the neuromas did not resolve after severe trimming it seems that there is critical amount of beak tissue that can be removed, beyond which neuromas will not resolve but will persist to adulthood.

The method of trimming can also influence the amount of tissue removed. The heat of cauterisation (approximately 700°C) can exacerbate damage to the beak stump, effectively increasing the amount of tissue removed at trimming (Breward and Gentle 1985; Lunam *et al.,* 1996). Excessive removal of beak tissue can result in a range of deformities following beak regrowth. These include abnormal focal swellings, splitting, a failure of the epidermis to regenerate resulting in chronic abrasion of the dermis and beak die-back, a condition in which the beak stump continues to degenerate.

Re-trimming

The effect of re-trimming on the formation and resolution of neuromas has been investigated in the chicken (Lunam *et al.,* 1998). In this study, beaks were moderately trimmed (half the upper and one-third of the lower beak) on the day of hatch. Some of the trimmed birds were randomly selected and were re-trimmed by removal of 2mm at 14 weeks-of-age. Neuromas were marginally more extensive after re-trimming. Although single trimmed and re-trimmed upper beaks had microneuromas at 14 and 28 (Figure 4.5A) and 66 weeks, these were less extensive with age indicative of long-term active resorption of the neuroma mass. A similar resolution of neuromas occurred in the lower beak with age. Re-trimming had no apparent affect on the ability of the neuroma to resorb as neuromas were absent in all lower beaks at 66 weeks-of-age. Similarly, re-trimming had no affect on behaviour in the long-term compared to the single trimming (Glatz *et al.*, 1998).

Concluding remarks

That neuromas persist in some beaks and that behaviours consistent with altered pain thresholds have been observed indicate that neuromas may evoke abnormal and painful stimuli. Caution however, needs to be applied in the interpretation of the presence or absence of neuromas in terms of welfare of the bird. Further work on physiology, behaviour and anatomy, in particular at the level of the spinal cord, needs to be undertaken in order to clarify the role of neuromas in chronic pain and altered pain thresholds after beak-trimming.

Acknowledgements

The author's research has been supported by grants from the Rural Industries Research and Development Corporation, the Egg Industry Research and Development Council, the Australian Research Council, the Flinders Medical Centre Research Foundation, the Flinders University Research Budget and the Flinders Medical Research Institute. I thank Dr Jenny Hiscock for her comments on this chapter and Kristy Weir for assistance with its preparation.

5

Physiological and behavioural aspects of beak-trimming in poultry

Ellen C. Jongman and John L. Barnett

Introduction

The incidence of aggressive pecking is generally fairly low in young birds, and increases as birds mature. Feather pecking and cannibalism are partly influenced by hormonal changes around the point of lay, when these behaviours can increase (Keeling 1995).

While beak-trimming decreases the damage caused by feather pecking it does not decrease the incidence of aggressive interactions, including feather pecking (Lee and Craig 1991; Craig, Winkler and Milliken 1992). However it does reduce the efficiency of pecking and thus the damage caused (Blokhuis and Van Der Haar 1989). There is a lot of opposition to beak-trimming on welfare grounds. However there is good indication that while beak-trimming results in short term pain, pullets with intact beaks may be under greater stress caused by painful aggressive interactions, indicated by higher corticosterone levels and changes in organ weights (Eskeland 1981; Struwe, Gleaves, Douglas and Bond 1992a; Struwe, Gleaves and Douglas 1992b). Depending on the criteria used it can both be argued that beak-trimming is stressful and affects welfare in a negative sense as well as the opposite, that beak-trimming alleviates stress caused by aggressive interactions (Lee and Craig 1991). This aspect of welfare assessment, which is essential to the interpretation of the behavioural and physical data on beak-trimming, is expanded upon in the next section.

Although removing as little as one-quarter of the beak is effective in reducing beak inflicted deaths (Kuo, Craig and Muir 1991) the removal of half of the beak in the same study was more effective in reducing deaths, while neither prevented beak inflicted deaths altogether. Good practice indicates that beak-trimming should be performed at hatch or soon after.

Many authors have reported a general suppression in activity after beak-trimming, lasting from 3 to 56 weeks, depending on age and severity of the trim. Lee and Graig (1990) observed that pullets trimmed at 4 weeks pecked less at food and their environment. They also stood and crouched more, were less active and showed more comfort behaviour than the control birds with intact beaks. Eskeland (1981) also found that hens trimmed at 18 weeks were less active. Duncan, Slee, Seawright and Breward (1989) confirmed that hens trimmed at 16 weeks were less active. This general reduction in activity may indicate the presence of pain, as the duration of reduced activity appears to coincide with the reduction in feed intake.

The Brambell Committee (1965) report on welfare objected to the practice of beak-trimming and recommended that it should be prohibited immediately in caged birds and within two years in birds kept on deep litter. Nearly forty years later beak-trimming is still common practice, although improvements in beak-trimming practices may have reduced the impact on the welfare of the birds over time. This chapter examines the current knowledge on the consequences of beak-trimming on behaviour as well as some physiological aspects. To assist in putting the findings in context this chapter also includes a section on welfare assessment (Barnett and Hemsworth 2003).

Welfare assessment

In science several definitions of animal welfare are in use. The following definition of Broom and Johnson (1993) is most widely used: The welfare of an individual is its state as regards its attempts to cope. In this definition, the "state as regards its attempts to cope" refers to both how much has to be done by the animal in order to cope with the environment and the extent to which the animal's coping attempts are succeeding. Attempts to cope include the functioning of body repair systems, immunological defences, physiological stress responses and a variety of behavioural responses. The risks to the welfare of an animal by an environmental challenge therefore can be assessed at two levels: firstly the magnitude of the behavioural and physiological responses and secondly the biological cost of these responses (Barnett and Hutson 1987; Broom and Johnson 1993; Hemsworth and Coleman 1998). These behavioural and physiological responses include the stress response while the biological cost includes adverse effects on the animal's ability to grow, reproduce and remain healthy.

It is generally accepted that there are three broad approaches used by scientists in studying animal welfare: the "feelings-based", the "nature of the species" and the "functioning-based" approaches (Duncan and Fraser 1997) also called the "homeostasis" approach. A fourth approach, the "animal preferences" approach, is sometimes included in the feelings approach but does not necessarily provide direct information on feelings or emotions. This approach involves studying the animal's choice for resources. Yet another approach is that based on the 'Five-Freedoms'. The starting point for the Five Freedoms was the UK Report of the Brambell Committee (1965) which concluded, amongst other things, that all intensively housed animals should be provided with sufficient space to be able to stand up, lie down, turn around, groom themselves and stretch. With developments over subsequent years, such behavioural requirements became known as the Five Freedoms. The UK Farm Animal Welfare Council proposed in 1992 that the welfare of animals can be protected by recognising the Five Freedoms (FAWC, 1992): 1) freedom from hunger and thirst, 2) freedom from discomfort, 3) freedom from pain, injury and disease, 4) freedom to express normal behaviour, 5) freedom from fear and distress.

The advantage of the "homeostasis" approach is that it contains some widely accepted criteria of poor welfare such as health, immunology, injuries and growth rate and nitrogen balance. Furthermore, there are some excellent examples of the value of this "homeostasis" approach in assessing animal welfare (Hemsworth and Coleman 1998). For example, handling studies on pigs have shown that fearful pigs have a sustained elevation of plasma free corticosteroid concentrations (Hemsworth and Barnett 1991; Hemsworth, Barnett and Hansen 1981; Hemsworth, Barnett and Hansen 1986a). The consequences of this chronic stress response in these fearful animals included depressions in growth and reproductive performance (Hemsworth *et al.,* 1981; Hemsworth *et al.,* 1986a; Hemsworth and Barnett 1991).

However, some of the subtler or less serious risks to welfare may not be detected by this method. Nevertheless, less serious challenges should be reflected in biological changes, although of lower magnitude, with consequent effects on fitness variables such as growth, reproduction, injury and health. Short-term challenges can also be studied with this approach. Lay, Friend, Grissom, Bowers and Mal (1992) studied the behavioural and physiological responses of cattle to two branding procedures to assess the relative aversiveness of the procedures and Hemsworth, Barnett and Campbell (1996) utilised behavioural and physiological responses together with growth performance to assess the welfare implications of a husbandry procedure regularly imposed (daily injections) on pigs.

The "homeostasis" approach appears to offer science the best assessment of the welfare of animals. As a research tool, this approach involves comparing housing or husbandry systems and risks to welfare are assessed on the basis of relative changes in biological (behavioural and physiological) responses and corresponding decreases in fitness. This is the approach used to assess welfare in this chapter. For a more complete discussion of welfare assessment, readers are referred to Barnett and Hemsworth (2003).

Effect on feed intake and pecking efficiency

Objections to the use of beak-trimming include its removal of sensory receptors, with a subsequent reduction in feed intake (Glatz and Lunam 1994), pecking efficiency (Gentle, Hughes and Hubrecht 1982) and pecking preferences (Hausberger 1992a; Hausberger 1992b).

Generally beak-trimming causes a temporarily reduction in feed intake and a reduced weight gain. However, beak-trimmed birds generally have improved feed efficiency (Bell and Adams 1998) and over time body weights of beak-trimmed birds return to or approach a normal weight range for intact birds (Carey 1990; Craig *et al.,* 1992).

Reduced feed intake after beak-trimming may indicate either pain associated with pecking or difficulty in eating after the removal of sensory receptors and an altered shape of the beak. Indeed, Gentle *et al.* (1982) found that hens trimmed during the laying period needed five times as many pecks to consume the same amount of feed in the form of pellets compared to intact controls. The increased number of pecks per gram of food may indicate that beak-trimmed pullets have reduced mechano-reception ability as a result of the altered beak shape. However when pullets were fed mash a reduction in feed intake after beak-trimming was not evident (Craig *et al.,* 1992). Workman and Rogers (1990) also found a reduction in feed intake due to decreased pecking efficiency. However, they also considered that food consumption may have been less rewarding due to a decrease of sensory feedback from the beak and this may have contributed to the reduction in feed intake.

Tanaka and Yoshimoto (1985) observed that many feed pecks made by laying hens are without the actual intent to eat. They regarded all pecks at food without eating as play eating. The increase in pecking at food while reducing feed consumption after beak-trimming may partly be explained as a result of phantom sensations or an increased stimulation of the beak.

Generally feed intake and body weight return to normal levels at the point of lay in birds trimmed early in life. This does not necessarily mean that the consequences of beak-trimming have disappeared since birds would be highly motivated to eat, as it is essential for survival.

Effect on sensory receptors

The beak is very versatile and highly sensitive, important for touch, temperature and nociceptive information. Beak-trimming results in permanent loss of temperature and touch responses because the sensory receptors do not regenerate when the beak re-grows (Gentle 1986b; Cunningham 1992). Gentle, Hughes, Fox and Waddington (1997) concluded that mild or moderate trimming at a young age resulted in significant regrowth of the beak. However it was not the shape or size of the beak that made beak-trimming an effective remedy against feather pecking and cannibalism but the permanent removal of sensory receptors at the tip of the beak (Gentle *et al.*, 1997). This was confirmed by Kuo *et al.* (1991) who found that when one-quarter of the beak was removed at 4 weeks-of-age the beak was fully regrown by the time the birds were 16 weeks-old. However there was still a significant reduction in beak related deaths, indicating that altered sensory reception may have been responsible for the reduction in cannibalistic pecking.

Beak-trimming may alter the sensory perception of the bird (Gentle *et al.*, 1982). The altered dimensions of the beak and the lack of sensory receptors in the beak may affect the accuracy of aiming at specific areas. It appears that this can result in both a decrease in the number of pecks made to the environment (Gentle, Waddington, Hunter and Jones 1990) as well as an increase in toe pecks and pecks made at the cage (Glatz, Lunam, Barnett and Jongman 1998). In this last study however, total number of pecks at the environment and at the feed was similar between trimmed and non-trimmed birds. This discrepancy between the two studies can partly be explained by the different ages when the birds were observed. Gentle *et al.* (1990) made their behavioural assessment 6 weeks after beak-trimming, whereas the observations by Glatz *et al.* (1998) were made 10 weeks after beak-trimming when the beak was healed and less chronic pain may be anticipated. Beak-trimming reduces litter directed behaviour (Blokhuis and Van Der Haar 1989; Sandilands and Savory 2002) but Sandilands and Savory (2002) found that trimmed birds spend more time preening directed at the preening gland. In contrast, Van Liere (1995) found that birds trimmed at 6 weeks-of-age showed a reduced responsiveness to a novel preening stimulus at 42 weeks. This indicates that beak-trimming has long lasting consequences on the use of the beak, which may affect the welfare of the bird.

Human amputees report not only phantom pain and stump pain, but also report phantom sensations (the feeling that the amputated limb is still present, (Jensen, Krebs, Nielsen and Rasmussen 1984; Jensen and Rasmussen 1994)). While birds may experience chronic pain after beak-trimming it is also possible that birds may experience phantom sensations. Perhaps the discrepancy of the sensations of the tip of an intact and a trimmed beak increases a type of investigative behaviour resulting in the increase of some pecking behaviour seen in several studies. Another explanation may be that beak-trimming results in a mild irritation rather than severe pain. Mild irritation may result in a mild stimulation of the beak (i.e toe pecks and cage pecks) persisting at a low but detectable level (Broom and Johnson 1993).

Evidence of pain

Pain caused by beak-trimming can be divided into immediate pain caused by the procedure itself and acute pain lasting for up to 15 to 30 days in older birds (refer Chapter 3) as damaged tissue heals. It is also possible that beak-trimming causes chronic pain lasting weeks or months as tissue heals and neuromas are formed, possibly resulting in 'stump pain' or phantom pain.

The beak contains both mechano-receptors and nociceptors and birds commonly struggle and vocalise during trimming especially when a hot blade is used (Grigor, Hughes and Gentle 1995). Gentle (1992) however reported that hens trimmed at 18 weeks remained immobile, much like the tonic immobility response to a stressor that cannot be avoided. It is not clear if birds that show the tonic immobility response feel pain, as this response is associated with an analgesic effect (Hutson, Curzon and Trickleband 1984). It is possible that this analgesic effect may last several hours after beak-trimming. Gentle *et al.* (1991) observed that there was no reduction in the number of pecks of birds 6 hours after beak-trimming, but a clear increase was seen 26 hours after trimming when the birds were again observed. Indeed, similar observations are made in people who show a pain-free period following full-thickness burns (Robertson, Cross and Terry 1985).

That pain is evident for at least a week after beak-trimming and up to 5 weeks is indicated by several behavioural changes. The skill of the operator when beak-trimming is very important, resulting in increased mortality if not carried out correctly. As mentioned earlier feed intake is reduced during the first few weeks after trimming, and although there may be several explanations for this, pain is likely to play a role. Several authors have reported greater inactivity in beak-trimmed birds, also a possible indication of pain (Duncan *et al.,* 1989; Lee and Craig 1990). A reduction in environmental pecking suggests guarding behaviour of a painful site, and was seen by Gentle *et al.* (1990) up to 6 weeks after trimming.

However, pain may persist for many weeks or even months. These aspects have been discussed in Chapter 3 but it is worth emphasing that chronic pain involves different mechanisms than acute pain. Pathological changes in the peripheral nervous system and physiological changes at the spinal cord and higher levels of the nervous system are implicated (Gentle 1992). Several authors found evidence of the formation of neuromas after beak-trimming (Lunam, Glatz and Hsu 1996) and abnormal spontaneous firing of afferent fibres (Breward and Gentle 1985). In humans neuromas and spontaneous firing of afferent fibres are associated with phantom pain or stump pain, but only a proportion of human patients experience chronic pain following amputation (Wall 1981). Changes in pain thresholds may also indicate the presence of chronic pain. In animals and man, it has been commonly found that thresholds to painful stimuli change in response to pain (Ley, Livingstone and Waterman 1989; Moiniche, Dahl and Kehlet 1993; Ley, Waterman and Livingstone 1995) and that this change indicates alterations in nerve function or nociceptive processing at higher levels (spinal cord or cerebral cortex). Glatz *et al*. (1998) found an increase in headshakes in beak-trimmed birds after drinking hot water at the pain threshold level (45°C). Headshakes may indicate a pain response after the beak is submerged in hot water (Gentle *et al.,* 1990). Whether the increased sensitivity to a painful stimulus was a result of changes in threshold of the pain receptors *per se* or a result of chronic pain remains unknown.

The above information on pain is based on beak-trimming conducted by the hot-blade technique (see Chapter 1). The behavioural and physical consequences of more recent methods such as infrared and laser are unknown.

Effect of age and re-trimming

It appears that the age of the bird at the time of beak-trimming affects the changes in behaviour. There is also evidence that there is less development of neuromas or even absence of neuromas and scar tissue in birds trimmed on day one or in the first few days of life (Desserich, Ziswiler and Folsch 1983; Desserich, Folsch and Ziswiler 1984). Duncan *et al*. (1989) found a reduction in preening and pecking 5 weeks after 16 week-old birds were trimmed and Gentle *et al*. (1990) found less pecking and drinking 6 weeks after trimming at 16 weeks. Eskeland (1981) even found suppression of activity lasting more than 56 weeks in birds that were trimmed at 18 weeks. In contrast Gentle *et al*. (1997) indicated that all differences in behaviour had disappeared 5 weeks after 1-day and 10-day old birds were trimmed.

Gentle *et al.* (1997) also noted rapid healing and no scar tissue at 21 and 45 days after trimming. It even appeared that effects of trimming were less in birds trimmed at 1-day old compared to birds at 10-day old, however confounding conditions during the experiment may have contributed to these differences. Beak-trimming at hatch may also be less stressful or painful than trimming at 10 and 42 days of age since Glatz *et al.* (1994) found no response in heart rate in chickens trimmed at hatch, while older birds showed an increase in heart rate in response to handling and beak-trimming. However, there was no difference in heart rate response between sham-trimmed and beak-trimmed birds at any age, indicating that handling in itself is quite stressful and that heart rate may not be a good measure of the additional stress or pain of beak-trimming itself. Hatching itself may be stressful and increase heart rate, explaining the lack of increase in heart rate during handling and beak-trimming.

When birds are trimmed early in life and no more than half of the beak is removed considerable regrowth occurs. It is common practice to re-trim these birds before point of lay to avoid feather pecking and cannibalism. Since only a small part of the beak is removed during re-trimming and no sensory receptors are removed (none have reappeared at the tip of the beak) very little effect of re-trimming is seen either on behaviour (Craig *et al.,* 1992; Glatz *et al.,* 1998) or neuroma formation (Glatz *et al.,* 1998).

Effect in turkeys

Although the majority of turkeys are not beak-trimmed, beak-trimming occurs in breeding stock and turkeys kept in more extensive systems When turkey beaks are trimmed early, healing appears to be rapid with no visible scarring or formation of neuromas (Gentle, Thorp and Hughes 1995).

Beak-trimming in one-day old tom turkeys does not appear to affect body weight and feed efficiency. Mortality as a consequence of cannibalism was reduced by beak-trimming although aggressive behaviour was not affected (Denbow, Leighton Jr. and Hulet 1984). In a similar study in female turkeys trimmed at 1-day old a reduction in feed intake and body weight gain was found at 16 weeks-of-age, but beak-trimming had no effect on any other measurements, including feather score. However the incidence of social pecking, and pecking and pulling of feathers, was increased in beak-trimmed birds, possibly due to inefficient use of the beak (Leighton Jr., Denbow and Hulet 1985).

Beak-trimming may have variable affects on different strains of turkeys. In a study that compared two commercial strains it was found that body weight and feed efficiency were improved by beak-trimming in both strains (Noble, Muir, Krueger and Nestor 1994). Although beak-trimming did not affect mortality in either strain, beak inflicted injuries were reduced in the strain that tended to have high levels of these injuries. This suggests that from a welfare perspective beak-trimming in turkeys should only occur in strains that show high levels of cannibalistic pecking.

Conclusions

Most effects of beak-trimming on behaviour and feed intake appear to be only short lasting, with beak-trimmed birds returning to normal levels within 3 to 5 weeks. Birds that are trimmed during the first few days of life return to normal behaviour more quickly than birds that are trimmed close to the start of lay. A moderate beak-trim early in life results in less body weight gain immediately after trimming, however most birds appear to approach normal body weight at the time of lay. When beak-trimming is more severe or later in life, body weights may be reduced long term. However, a moderate trim early in life may result in considerable regrowth and may necessitate re-trimming before point of lay, although re-trimming does not appear to result in chronic pain. The formation of neuromas, and possibly chronic pain, also appear greatly diminished if birds are trimmed early in life. For an over view of the effects of beak-trimming on behaviour and physiological responses see Table 5.1.

At present beak-trimming appears to be necessary to limit stress in birds that may otherwise be subject to excessive pecking. However, there is a lack of comprehensive studies that measure the effect of beak-trimming on welfare using multiple indicators (physiological as well as behavioural) and it is hard to compare between studies due to different methods of beak-trimming and beak-trimming at different ages. Although much of the literature indicates that beak-trimming itself results in chronic pain, modern practice of trimming at an early age and limiting the amount of beak that is removed appear to reduce the incidence and duration of chronic pain. With the development of new and better techniques such as infrared and laser, chronic pain may be even further reduced or avoided all together. Nevertheless, beak-trimming will always cause a deprivation of sensory input of the beak, an important source of information in birds, and the end goal should be the avoidance of beak-trimming altogether through genetics, housing conditions and management.

Table 5.1 Summary of possible behavioural and physiological responses as a result of beak-trimming.

Behaviour and physiological changes	Reference
Behavioural response during beak-trim procedure, indicative of pain and stress. Behavioural response can vary from struggle and vocalisation to a tonic immobility response.	Grigor et al. 1995; Gentle 1992
Reduced general activity, which may be indicative of pain.	Lee and Craig, 1990; Eskeland, 1981; Duncan et al. 1989
Reduced pecking efficiency, with more pecks at food needed to achieve the same food intake and may lead to reduced feed intake.	Gentle et al. 1982; Workman and Rogers, 1990
Reduced feed intake, possibly caused by pain and/or reduced pecking efficiency.	Glatz and Lunam, 1994; Workman and Rogers, 1990
Loss of sensory receptors, which will affect pecking behaviour and use of the beak	Cunningham, 1992; Gentle, 1986b; Gentle et al. 1990; Glatz et al. 1998; Gentle, Hughes, Fox and Waddington, 1997; Gentle et al. 1982; Blokhuis and Van der Haar, 1989; Sandilands and Savory, 2002; Vanliere, 1995
Permanent neurological changes, including forming of neuromas, abnormal spontaneous firing of afferent nerves as well as changes at the higher levels of the nervous system.	Lunam, Glatz and Hsu, 1996; Breward and Gentle, 1985; Gentle, 1992
Changes in pain thresholds of the beak.	Glatz et al. 1998; Gentle et al. 1990

6

Production responses of beak-trimmed birds

Patricia Y. Hester

Introduction

Beak-trimming effects on performance parameters of domesticated chickens have been researched extensively (Gentle 1986b; Cunningham 1992; Mench 1992; Cunningham and Mauldin 1996; Hester and Shea-Moore 2003). Production characteristics often evaluated in beak-trimming studies include liveability, feed intake, body weight, feed efficiency, feathering condition, age at sexual maturity, egg production, egg weight and egg quality. The age and severity of beak-trimming greatly affect performance traits. In addition, production parameters among strains and breeds of poultry do not always respond in a similar manner to beak-trimming (Craig and Lee 1990).

Liveability

In the majority of studies reported to date, liveability among White Leghorns during the pullet phase is similar between beak-trimmed and beak-intact flocks (Andrade and Carson 1975; Sundaresen, Jayaprasad and Kothandaraman 1979; Lee 1980; Deaton, Lott, Branton and Simmons 1987; Carey 1990). An exception occurred with ISA Browns in which cannibalism between 17 and 20 weeks-of-age caused a dramatic increase in pre-lay mortality in untrimmed birds as compared to those whose beaks were trimmed at 10 weeks-of-age by removing 1.0 cm of the upper beak and 0.5 cm of the lower beak (Hartini, Choct, Hinch, Kocher and Nolan 2002). While pullet mortality is generally unaffected by beak-trimming, at least in White Leghorns, substantial data show that laying house liveability is improved in beak-trimmed flocks when compared to beak intact flocks (Carson 1975; Lee and Reid 1977; Lee 1980; Eskeland 1981; Craig and Lee 1990; Kuo, Craig and Muir 1991; Lee and Craig 1991; Maizama and Adams 1994; Anderson and Davis 1997; Hartini *et al.*, 2002). Mortality, as a result of beak-inflicted injuries, is generally reduced as a greater portion of the beak is trimmed (Kuo *et al.*, 1991).

Feed intake and body weight

When beak-trimming is done at an early age, feed intake and body weights are reduced (Blokhuis, Van Der Haar and Koole 1987; Bell and Kuney 1991; Glatz and Lunam 1994; Gentle, Hughes, Fox and Waddington 1997; Hartini *et al.,* 2002) however, by the time chickens reach sexual maturity or peak egg production, growth rates return to normal (Hargreaves and Champion 1965; Beane, Siegel and Dawson 1967; Andrade and Carson 1975; Lee and Reid 1977; Lee 1980; Carey 1990; Craig and Lee 1990; Lee and Craig 1990; Lee and Craig 1991; Struwe, Gleaves and Douglas 1992b). When greater proportions of beaks of hens are trimmed when hens are producing eggs, feed intake and body weight are reduced. For example, removal of 4, 6, and 8 mm of the beak of adult hens caused a decrease in feed intake and body weight (Glatz 1987). Removal of less of the beak (3 mm) of egg laying chickens at 38 weeks-of-age also exhibited depressed feed intake for 9 to 10 days following the trim, but by 42 weeks-of-age body weights were not affected. A more moderate trim in which only 2 mm of the beak of 38 week-old hens is removed did not affect feed intake. Gentle, Hughes and Hubrecht (1982) also reported a reduction in feed intake and body weight when adult hens had half, but not one-third, of their beaks trimmed. Collectively, these results suggest that unlike severe trims, a mild trimming of beaks of hens in egg production does not affect feed consumption and body weight.

Feed efficiency

Beak-trimmed pullets (Sundaresen *et al.,* 1979) and laying hens (Slinger and Pepper 1964; Lee and Reid 1977; Lee 1980; Maizama and Adams 1994; Anderson and Davis 1997) have improved feed efficiencies when compared to beak intact controls. Feed wastage has been suggested as one possible reason for the increased feed usage noted in beak intact controls (Bauermann 1959; Sundaresen *et al.,* 1979; Blokhuis *et al.,* 1987; Glatz 1990). In a study by Craig, Craig and Milliken (1992), they actually documented that feed usage by beak-trimmed White Leghorns was 18% less than beak intact controls. Feed usage per day, which included feed consumed and feed wasted, averaged 119 and 144 g for beak-trimmed and beak intact birds, respectively. Another factor possibly contributing to better feed efficiencies of beak-trimmed flocks is improved feather covering over non-trimmed flocks, thus decreasing requirements for maintenance (Hughes and Michie 1982).

Feather condition

Plumage quality is improved with beak-trimming, most likely due to reduced feather pulling and picking. Beak-trimming performed at 25 days-of-age with the cutting and cauterization of half of the upper beak and less of the bottom beak improved feather condition of White Leghorns at 36 weeks-of-age as compared to those birds whose beaks were left intact (Craig and Lee 1990; Lee and Craig 1991). Likewise, three strains of White Leghorn chickens maintained at Kansas State University in which half of the upper beak and less of the bottom beak was cut and cauterised at 24 days-of-age showed improved feathering at 20 and 21 weeks-of-age (Lee and Craig 1991). Anderson and Davis (1997) reported improved feather scores in caged Dekalb White Leghorns whose beaks were trimmed at 6 days (2.8 mm guide hole, quarter of the beak removed) and 11 weeks (2 mm of beak retained following trimming, two-thirds of the beak removed) when compared to beak intact controls. Beak intact pullets, as compared to pullets whose beaks were trimmed, demonstrated feather pecking causing bare spots on the backs of some birds. Cannibalism was also evident among beak intact birds at the end of the pullet growing period (Van Rooijen and Blokhuis 1990; Struwe *et al.,* 1992b). Feather pulling and picking was reduced by removing two-thirds of the beak at one day-of-age as compared to beak intact Leghorns (Lee and Reid 1977). By 80 weeks-of-age, the back, tail, and neck regions were bare in the untrimmed flock, and 6 of 200 beak intact birds had died of cannibalism due to severe pecking (Lee and Reid 1977). The plumage quality was improved in 78 week-old medium-bodied hens whose beaks were trimmed at 18 weeks-of-age as compared to beak intact controls (Hughes and Michie 1982). Both floor-reared and wire-reared birds demonstrated improved feather condition as a result of beak-trimming (Struwe, Gleaves, Douglas and Bond 1992a). These results clearly demonstrate that a benefit of beak-trimming is improved feather condition.

Age at sexual maturity

Chicks whose beaks are trimmed experience a short delay in sexual maturity (Slinger and Pepper 1964; Beane *et al.,* 1967; Andrade and Carson 1975; Lee and Reid 1977; Craig and Lee 1989; Kuo *et al.,* 1991). An exception is with a severe trim in which the entire upper beak from the nostrils to the tip is removed results in a substantial delay in sexual maturity (Hargreaves and Champion 1965). Kuo *et al.* (1991) concluded that the short delay in sexual maturation caused by moderate beak-trimming is likely to be inconsequential to total egg output (Figure 6.1).

Egg production

Moderate beak-trimming does not affect egg production (Table 6.1). A few reports indicate improved egg production in beak-trimmed hens as compared to beak intact controls (Morgan 1957; Eskeland, Bjornstad and Hvidsten

1977; Eskland 1981; Glatz 1990; Kuo *et al.,* 1991; Craig 1992). An impairment in egg production was noted when 18 week-old pullets were subjected to a severe trim in which the entire upper and lower beaks were removed from the tip to the nostrils (Hargreaves and Champion 1965).

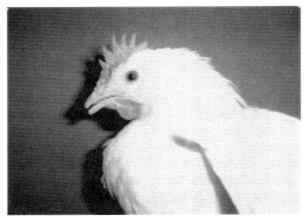

Figure 6.1 White Leghorn pullet subjected to a moderate beak-trim at hatch. A short delay in sexual maturity caused by beak-trimming is inconsequential to total egg output.

Egg quality and weight

Beak-trimming does not affect the thickness of the shell, the incidence of blood spots in eggs, or albumen height (Yannakopoulos and Tserven-Gousi 1986). Egg weight is generally not affected by beak-trimming (Hargreaves and Champion 1965; Yannakopoulos and Tserven-Gousi 1986; Craig and Lee 1989; Struwe *et al.,* 1992b; Anderson and Davis 1997), though there are some reports indicating a decrease in egg weight due to beak-trimming (Slinger and Pepper 1964; Lee 1980; Bell 1996).

Second beak-trim

Pullets are often subjected to a second trim between the ages of 5 and 12 weeks-of-age, especially when the initial trim is performed on hatchlings or on chicks prior to 10 days-of-age. A second trimming of the beak is more permanent in that subsequent regrowth of the beak is less likely. A second trim offers economic advantage to the producer in that feed usage is lowered without adversely affecting performance traits. In a study using two commercial strains of egg layers, Carey and Lassiter (1995) reported on the economic advantage of a second trim.   Chicks were initially trimmed at 10 days-of-age with a second trimming at either 9 or 12 weeks-of-age. Since

Table 6.1 The effect of beak-trimming on egg production.

Age of bird	Amount of beak removed	Breed	Egg production%		Reference
			Beak-trimmed	Beak intact	
1 day	1/3 upper and lower	New Hampshire	94.7*	77.0*	Morgan, 1957
1 day	1/2 upper	New Hampshire	90.3*	77.0*	Morgan, 1957
Various times during egg laying	1/2 upper, 4 mm of lower	White Leghorn	64.5	65.7	Bray et al. 1960
Various times during egg laying	1/2 upper, 4 mm of lower	White Leghorn	68.5	61.7	Bray et al. 1960
Various times during egg laying	1/2 upper, 4 mm of lower	White Rock	31.7	38.4	Bray et al. 1960
Various times during egg laying	1/2 upper, 4 mm of lower	Rhode Island Red	53.8	54.3	Bray et al. 1960
Various times during egg laying	1/2 upper, 4 mm of lower	New Hampshire	33.5	29.2	Bray et al. 1960
8 weeks	2/3 upper, 1/3 lower	White Leghorn	70.4	73.0	Slinger and Pepper, 1964
20 weeks	2/3 upper, 1/3 lower	White Leghorn	73.1	73.0	Slinger and Pepper, 1964
18 or 24 weeks	1/2 upper, less lower	White Leghorn	179[1]	188[1]	Hargreaves and Champion, 1965
18 or 24 weeks	3/4 upper, less lower	White Leghorn	173[1]	188[1]	Hargreaves and Champion, 1965
18 or 24 weeks	Entire upper trimmed, less lower	White Leghorn	127[1,*]	188[1,*]	Hargreaves and Champion, 1965
8 weeks	1/2 upper	White Leghorn	70.6	68.3	Cooper and Barnett, 1967
1 day	2/3 upper	White Leghorn	75.2	73.3	Lee and Reid, 1977

Table 6.1 Contd.

Age of bird	Amount of beak removed	Breed	Egg production% Beak-trimmed	Beak intact	Reference
1 day	2/3 upper	White Leghorn	68.9	67.1	Lee, 1980
4 weeks	2/3 upper	White Leghorn	70.2	67.1	Lee, 1980
8 weeks	2/3 upper	White Leghorn	71.3	67.1	Lee, 1980
18 weeks	1/3 upper	White Leghorn	57.5*	52.2*	Eskeland, 1981
18 weeks	1/3 upper	White Leghorn	69.5*	63.9*	Eskeland, 1981
18 days	No information	White Leghorn	82.0	85.3	Yannakopoulos and Tserven-Gousi, 1986
4 weeks	1/2 upper, less of lower	White Leghorn	74.3	73.7	Craig and Lee, 1989
1 day	1/2 upper and 1/3 lower	Australian brown and tinted egg strains	78.7*	73.3*	Glatz, 1990
10 days	1/2 upper and 1/3 lower	Australian brown and tinted egg strains	77.2*	73.3*	Glatz, 1990
42 days	1/2 upper and 1/3 lower	Australian brown and tinted egg strains	77.0*	73.3*	Glatz, 1990
4 weeks	1/4 upper, less of lower	White Leghorn	59.9	56.9	Kuo *et al.* 1991
4 weeks	1/2 upper, less of lower	White Leghorn	68.6*	56.9*	Kuo *et al.* 1991
10 days	2/3 upper and slightly less of lower	White Leghorn	83.1 *	81.3*	Craig, 1992
10 days	No information	White Leghorn	81.0	81.0	Struwe *et al.* 1992b
7 days	~1/3 upper	White Leghorn	75.8	75.4	Maizama and Adams, 1994
10 days	~1/3 upper	White Leghorn	77.9	75.4	Maizama and Adams, 1994
6 to 7 weeks	upper and lower	White Leghorn	69.3*	71.3*	Bell, 1996

*Indicates significant difference between beaked-trimmed and beak-intact birds.
[1]Data of Hargreaves and Champion (1965) expressed as average total egg production.

there were no beak intact controls in this study, the birds that were trimmed twice were compared to the single–trimmed birds. The second trimming resulted in reduced feed usage that persisted through the end of lay as compared to those birds that were only beak-trimmed at 10 days-of-age. Birds subjected to a second trim had egg production, egg weights, and feed efficiencies similar to single trimmed birds. If feed savings as a result of reduced feed usage could offset the labor costs associated with a second trim, then an economic incentive prevails to subject birds to a second trim (Carey and Lassiter 1995). In an earlier study, Carey (1990) compared the performance of three commercial egg laying strains that were beak-trimmed at 7 days-of-age with a second trim at 9, 12, and 15 weeks-of-age. Beak-intact controls or chicks only subjected to a single trim were not included in this study. Production performance results were similar to Carey and Lassiter (1995) with the exception that hens subjected to a second trim at 9 weeks-of-age experienced decreased egg production when compared to pullets receiving second trims at 12 and 15 weeks-of-age. Carey (1990) commented on the economic and welfare issues of a second beak-trim suggesting that an egg production loss of 1% experienced by birds given a second trim at 9 weeks-of-age could be offset by lower feed costs and mortality.

Kuney and Bell (1982) evaluated the effect of a second trim at 12 weeks-of-age using two strains of White Leghorns that were lightly beak-trimmed at 7 days-of-age. The second trim compared three methods: 1) a one-cut method in which both the upper and lower beak was trimmed simultaneously, 2) a moderate two-cut method in which two thirds of the upper beak followed by one-third of the lower beak were trimmed, and 3) a severe two-cut method in which two-thirds of both the upper and then the lower beak were trimmed. Beak intact controls or birds subjected to only a single trim were not used in this experiment. The best hen-day and hen-house egg production and feed efficiency were noted in birds subjected to the more severe final trim when compared to birds subjected to the other two beak-trimming methods.

Bell and Kuney (1991) revisited the effects of a second beak-trimming by comparing three commercial strains of White Leghorns that were subjected to a second trim at either 6 or 12 weeks-of-age. The first trim occurred at 10 days-of-age in which the upper beak of chicks was trimmed within 2 mm of the nostril, while the lower beak was trimmed slightly longer. The second trim at 6 or 12 weeks-of-age resulted in the removal of the upper beak within 4 and 5 mm of the nostril, respectively. The bottom beak was also subjected to a second trim and was 1 mm longer than the upper beak for trims at both 6 and 12 weeks-of-age. Hen-house and hen-day egg production, total egg mass, and total egg income were improved in hens given a second trim at 6 weeks-of-age as compared to hens given a second trim at 12 weeks-of-age.

Conclusions

Advantages of beak-trimming include improved liveability, plumage quality and feed efficiency during egg laying. Moderate beak-trimming at a young age does not detrimentally affect subsequent egg production and quality (Slinger and Pepper 1964; Yannakopoulos and Tserven-Gousi 1986; Carey and Lassiter 1995). Beak-trimming caused reduced feed usage and body weight during the pullet phase (Slinger, Pepper and Sibbald 1962; Hartini *et al.,* 2002) and, in some instances, the laying phase (Slinger and Pepper 1964), especially if birds were subjected to a second trim (Carey and Lassiter 1995). The reduction in feed usage and body weight of beak-trimmed birds are viewed by some researchers as an advantage rather than a disadvantage (Slinger *et al.,* 1962; Slinger and Pepper 1964; Andrade and Carson 1975; Carey and Lassiter 1995). Because feed cost represents a significant proportion of total production cost, beak-trimming has an economic advantage in net income as compared to non-trimmed controls (Anderson and Davis 1997). If birds are not beak-trimmed and are provided with a less competitive feeding environment because of increased cage and feeder space allocation (United Egg Producers, 2002), some strains of chickens may have to be subjected to timed feeding or mild feed restriction to achieve optimal body weights. However, using feed restriction to improve feed efficiency and control body weight may not improve well-being if hungry birds display increased pecking leading to cannibalism (Arulswaminathan 1996) or show any other deleterious physiological or behavioural responses. As with beak-trimming, there are labor costs associated with feed restriction programs. Moreover, managerial skills and close supervision are required for both beak-trimming and feed restriction to prevent mishaps. Equipment manufacturers may want to consider a redesign of feeders (Figure 6.2) to minimise feed wastage and improve feed usage by beak intact birds (Craig *et al.,* 1992).

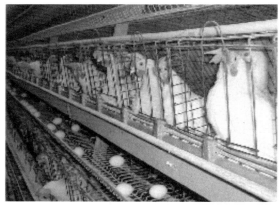

Figure 6.2 A redesign of feeder systems may be an option for future consideration by equipment manufacturers to reduce feed wastage by beak intact flocks.

7

Bird health and handling issues associated with beak-trimming

Philip C. Glatz and Zhihong H. Miao

Introduction

The health of birds after beak-trimming can be influenced by age, and method and severity of beak-trimming (Lunam, Glatz and Hsu 1996; Gentle, Hughes, Fox and Waddington 1997; Glatz, Lunam, Barnett and Jongman 1998; Hester and Shea-Moore 2003). Handling of birds for trimming is less stressful for birds at a younger age. The most popular age for beak-trimming in industry is 5-10 days-of-age because of reduced mortality and beak regrowth, but research indicates that day-old beak-trimming causes the least stress (Glatz 2000). This chapter outlines the problems associated with beak-trimming (Wells 1983) especially when it is not done correctly.

Physical damage to the birds while being handled for beak-trimming

The physical handling of the birds during beak-trimming should be done in a manner which avoids harm and damage to the birds. The major risks to birds are broken bones while being handled before and after beak-trimming. These risks can be minimised by careful handling. Day-old birds can be safely handled by picking them up by one hand and wrapping the fingers gently around the chest and abdomen. Birds can also be scooped with both hands cupped. Up to 4 chickens can be handled in this manner ensuring birds do not spill from the sides of the hand. For 7-10 day olds, birds can be picked up by one or two legs and transferred directly to the beak-trimmer located outside the pen. With 7-10 day olds, 5 chickens can be held in each hand. Alternatively birds can be gently pushed into a large laundry bucket held on an angle or placed into crates prior to beak-trimming. The Australian Code of Practice for Poultry (SCARM 1995) indicates that crates used to hold poultry before trimming should be of a design to prevent escape. In addition the protrusion of any part of a bird through the crate should be avoided such that it cannot become entrapped or damaged during handling.

Crates should be designed, monitored and managed such that birds are not injured when being placed in or taken out. Containers should be of a sufficient height to allow poultry to stand. Crates should not be tilted while still containing birds. Birds should not be held in crates for more than 24 h prior to beak-trimming (adapted from Bourke, Glatz, Barnett and Critchley 2002). If pullets are reared in cages they can be very flighty and extra care is needed when removing birds from the cage, especially when being re-trimmed at 8-12 weeks-of-age. Some will clutch the cage floor. These birds need to be held by both legs to loosen their grip on the cage floor. They should be handled and crated gently to avoid injury. At all times care should take precedence over speed and labour cost. Nevertheless birds still suffer from bone breakage when handled roughly. Birds should not be lifted or carried by the head, neck, tail or wing. When pullets are being handled for re-trimming it is recommended that no more than 10 birds (5 per hand) be carried, up to 2.0 kg of weight. This limit should also apply for birds being carried from the penning area to the beak-trimmer.

Pile-ups and suffocation through incorrect penning and handling procedures

When penning the birds throughout the catching process prior to trimming care needs to be taken to ensure that pile-ups and suffocation do not occur. When beak-trimming is being done on day-old birds in the hatchery they can be held in cardboard boxes with holes in the side or plastic trays. However, as the birds become older, the flight fear response increases. At 7-10 days-of-age when beak-trimming is normally done, birds will panic and try to escape. When re-trimming is done at 8-14 weeks the flight fear response is greater and many birds will attempt to escape. These birds require extra care when catching before being beak-trimmed. The shed lighting should be dimmed so that the birds do not over-react to any other influence particularly from staff movements in the shed. It is important for staff to move quietly and carefully through the shed with very slow movements and wear clothing that is familiar to the birds to reduce bird stress level. There should be no yelling or shouting at the birds because this causes them to panic. If there is no stress and panic in birds, the birds will be calmer and result in a better beak-trim. Before penning the birds prior to beak-trimming at 7-10 days or at 8-12 weeks it is advisable to use blue lights, as birds tend to remain calmer (adapted from Bourke et al., 2002). Stressors in practical poultry production situations (ammonia, beak-trimming, coccidiosis, intermittent electric shock) decrease the weight gain, feed intake and feed conversion efficiency (McFarlane, Curtis, Shanks and Carmer 1989). With few exceptions, each stressor affects hematologic, body composition and pathologic traits in a similar manner whether imposed singly or concurrently (McFarlane, Curtis, Simon and Izquierdo 1989). Ordinarily birds experience more than one stressor at the same time. Effects of the multiple concurrent unrelated stressors on performance may be estimable by summing effects of respective stressors when acting alone. McFarlane and Curtis (1989) reported that the chick's leukocyte changes in response to the stress were less variable and more enduring than its corticosterone response, and the heterophil:lymphocyte ratio was sometimes a more reliable indicator of stress.

Chickens should not be kept in confined surrounds for more than 15 min as they will overheat, especially in hot weather, and tend to bleed more readily when beak-trimmed. Wire mesh surrounds or catching frames are recommended, as they do not restrict the ventilation. Wire mesh should be covered with hessian to prevent stacking and pile-ups of birds. The Australian Code of Practice for Domestic Poultry (SCARM, 1995) states that birds should be herded for pick up only under the supervision of a competent person to avoid suffocation and bruising. They should be handled and crated gently to avoid injury (adapted from Bourke *et al.*, 2002).

Acute blood loss and death due to bleeding

Birds need to be trimmed and cauterised correctly and at the correct age during their primary beak-trim to avoid bleeding and in some cases to prevent severe blood loss leading to death. Bleeding usually occurs if the beak has not been cauterised properly or if the blade is too hot or cold. High temperature and stress in birds caused by rough handling (noise and yelling) also increases the number of bleeders (adapted from Bourke *et al.*, 2002). Birds that are bleeding after beak-trimming, attract the attention of other birds. It is also common for other birds to gently peck at the wound on beaks of other birds. This encourages birds at a later stage to initiate cannibalism especially after they have got the initial taste for blood. It is recommended to apply an extra 1 sec cauterisation to seal the wound. The beak can also be dipped in ice water soon after beak-trimming to cool the wound and prevent bleeding (adapted from Bourke *et al.*, 2002).

Severe check of birds growth due to restricted ability to drink (particularly from nipple drinkers)

Heidweiller, van Loon and Zweers (1992) studied the drinking mechanism in adult chickens. Most behaviour elements of the drinking mechanism were so flexible that a chicken could reorganize the movement patterns of jaws, tongue, larynx, and head to adapt the mechanism to beak-trimming changes. Although the rate of water intake in beak-trimmed chickens was about 35% lower compared to normal beak chickens due to longer beak immersion time, these chickens approached a drinker very carefully and rotated their heads to maximize the area of the bill tips that contacted the water. Tongue movements were readily adjusted to maximize water intake in different external conditions or after serious damage to the beak. There were also additional adaptive changes in head-neck patterning by beak-trimmed chickens.

Loss of flock uniformity and subsequent competitive starve outs

Vitamin D3 plays an important role in beak formation. Stevens, Blair, Salmon and Stevens (1984) found that beak malformations (mainly an underdeveloped top mandible) occurred in 49.5% of the dead embryos from hens fed 300 IU vitamin D3/kg feed. This variation could result in uneven flock development and may affect the production ability of the flock at a later stage. Some birds come into lay earlier than others and egg weight and other production parameters may be variable. The various combinations of inappropriate beak-trimming, feeder and drinker types and availability and stocking densities can lead to the most commonly observed problem after beak-trimming of loss of flock uniformity. This will result in overall poorer flock performance with lower peak production and less eggs per hen housed. If severe the flock may experience significant numbers of starve outs and the need to cull these chickens (P. Scott, pers. com.).

The method of beak-trimming affects the performance of the birds. With severe beak-trimming, the birds have difficulty eating and drinking and growth may be retarded. If insufficient beak is cut, the beak will quickly regrow and the beak needs to be trimmed again. If the beak cut is in an improper angle, the beak can become deformed (Shirley 1977).

Secondary Staphylococcal infection in damaged beaks

Beak-trimming should only be done by an accredited beak-trimmer or by a trainee under appropriate supervision. Following beak-trimming, there is regrowth of the keratin layers. The cut end heals and is recovered with the keratin beak tissues. In some cases, however, the keratin layers may not be able to regrow enough for the cut surface to recover. In this situation fibrous tissue (softer than keratin) covered by an epithelial layer abrades and erodes, leaving a surface that is granulated with a permanent scab. Many birds manage to eat and perform normally with this wound but the open nature of the lesion can provide an entry point for bacteria. This typically produces a local infection manifesting as fibromatous lumps on the face, which when incised contain caseous material (K. Critchley, pers. com). Likewise if the cauterisation is inadequate, there is also potential for bacteria to enter in through the cut and cause an infection (adapted from Bourke *et al.*, 2002). In some cases the type of feeder and drinker can lead to continued irritation of the recently trimmed beak resulting in this area of the beak acting as a portal of entry for bacteria such as *Staphylococcus* spp.

Distorted (twisted) beak with feed prehension problems.

If the beak-trimming is done improperly, distorted beaks can occur. For example, when the blade is too cold, the operator may believe that they have cauterised the beak but when pulling the beak away from the blade they tear the beak. This can also cause bulbous type growths on the beak (adapted from Bourke *et al.*, 2002).

Secondary Marek's outbreaks after beak-trimming

Lee (1980) found that mortality of laying hens was significantly reduced with Marek's disease (MD) vaccination (cell-free herpesvirus of turkey) and day-old beak-trimming (removing about two-thirds of upper beak with an electric debeaker at day-old, 4 weeks or 8 weeks). Similar result were reported by Lee and Reid (1977). However, this effect was not significant for growing birds indicating that an out-break of MD and severe cannibalism are not present during the growing period. However, if flocks that are marginally vaccinated for MD, undergo other immunosuppressive illnesses or environmental challenge with Marek's virus, clinical levels of MD may occur shortly after trimming older birds, eg. around 12 weeks-of-age (P. Scott, pers. com.).

Conclusion

The physical handling of the birds during beak-trimming should be done in a manner which avoids harm and damage to the birds. The major risks to birds are broken bones while being handled before and after beak-trimming. These risks can be minimised by careful handling. Day-old birds can be safely handled by picking them up by one hand and wrapping the fingers gently around the chest and abdomen.

When penning the birds throughout the catching process prior to trimming care needs to be taken to ensure that pile-ups and suffocation do not occur. Birds need to be trimmed and cauterised correctly and at the correct age during their primary beak-trim to avoid bleeding and in some cases to prevent severe blood loss leading to death.

With severe beak-trimming, the birds have difficulty eating and drinking and growth may be retarded. If insufficient beak is cut, the beak will quickly regrow and the beak needs to be trimmed again. If the beak cut is in an improper angle, the beak can become deformed.

8

Alternatives to beak-trimming

Alternatives to beak-trimming - Foreword

Following growing public concern, conventional battery cages will be banned throughout the European Community from 2012. However, although furnished cages (containing perches, nest boxes, dust baths) will still be allowed, the potentially significant uptake of supposedly more 'animal-friendly' alternative systems, like aviaries or free range, may engender their own set of welfare problems. Feather pecking, which describes one bird pecking at and pulling out the feathers of another, is a prime example. Apart from imposing an economic burden, (e.g. because denuded birds need to eat more in order to keep warm), it can cause pain (see Chapter 3) and it may lead to cannibalism (see Chapter 1) and the painful, protracted death of target birds. Feather pecking is particularly problematic in alternative systems because it is much more difficult to control this behavioural vice when the birds (laying hens, broiler breeders, ducks, pheasants, turkeys, guinea fowl) are kept in the large flocks common to such systems. Currently, the remedial measures that are used to alleviate feather pecking include beak-trimming and/or keeping the birds under very dim light. However, these treatments can cause chronic pain (see Chapter 3) and eye abnormalities, respectively. Furthermore, the UK's Farm Animal Welfare Council considered "that beak-trimming is a most undesirable mutilation which should be avoided if at all possible" (FAWC, 1997). Clearly, the timely identification of practical, effective and affordable alternative methods of minimising this harmful behaviour is essential. There are a number of nutritional, management, environmental enrichment and selective breeding strategies that can be used as an alternative to beak-trimming.

These alternatives to beak-trimming are outlined in the subsequent sections.

R. Bryan Jones

8.1

Environmental enrichment can reduce feather pecking

R. Bryan Jones

Introduction

Effective environmental enrichment should expand the repertoire of desirable behaviours, reduce the occurrence of harmful ones, sustain the animals' long-term interest, and enable them to cope with challenges more adaptively. Traditionally, enrichment has involved increasing environmental complexity and thereby encouraging the animal to interact with its home environment. This is normally achieved by introducing various objects, biological materials, pictures, foods, sounds and/or odours into chickens' cages or floor pens (Jones 2001; Jones 2002). This has been reported to reduce fearfulness, boredom and feather pecking (Jones 2002). The provision of cage furniture, like nest boxes, perches and dust baths, may also help to satisfy some of the birds' behavioural requirements but, for present purposes, this section will focus on attempts to develop simple enrichment devices that sustain interest and divert injurious pecking away from flock mates.

Developing practical enrichment devices to minimise feather pecking

A wide range of objects has been used to provide putative enrichment for chickens (Jones 2001). Several stimuli were introduced simultaneously into the birds' cages in most studies but this made it difficult to ascribe any beneficial effects that may have been observed to specific stimuli. Furthermore, the birds ignored many of these so-called enrichment stimuli and some combinations of devices were actually associated with increased aggression. This probably reflected the fact that they had been chosen according to human preconceptions of environmental enrichment rather than a critical assessment of the birds' preferences.

To the best of knowledge, only three types of 'enrichment stimuli' have been tested in isolation. First, the Agrotoy (Gallus Ltd., Israel), which consisted of a blue plastic 7.5 x 5.0 cm frame with a red hanger on which were attached red and blue moving parts, was reported to reduce aggressiveness and mortality in caged laying hens (Gvaryahu, Ararat, Asaf, Lev, Weller, Robinson and Snapir 1994). Second, a small silver bell was found to attract significantly more pecking over a 2-week period than the Agrotoy (Gao, Feddes and Robinson 1994), but bird behaviour and mortality were not recorded in this study. Third, incorporating Peckablocks (Breckland International Ltd., England) which consist of a 18 x 7 cm, cereal-based enrichment device, in the pens of growing broiler chicks was claimed to reduce the amount of aggressive behaviour directed at other birds (Guy 2001). However, these devices do not appear to be in widespread use.

For these reasons, and following behavioural observations of birds at commercial farms, a series of experiments was carried out to systematically assess chickens' pecking preferences for selected stimuli. These experiments (Jones, Carmichael and Rayner 2000; Jones 2001; Jones 2002; Jones and Ruschak 2002) revealed that both chicks and adult laying hens pecked sooner and much more often at bunches of plain white string (polypropylene baling twine) than at all the other stimuli that were tested; these included beads, baubles, chains, feathers, and a commercially available device (PECKA-BLOCK). In addition to the pecking and pulling that was directed at all the stimuli, the birds teased apart the strands of the string in a way that resembled preening. Thus, its greater attractiveness may have reflected the fact that it seemed to provide the most positive feedback.

The string devices consisted of 4 or 8 lengths of white polypropylene twine each measuring either 16 x 0.5, 32 x 0.5 or 48 x 0.5 cm (length x diameter) for chicks, growing birds and adult hens, respectively. These were doubled over and a length of nylon fishing line was passed between the lengths at the mid point, which was then bound with white tape (Figure 8.1.1). The fishing line can then be used to secure the string device to the roof of the cage, to a perch or to another suitable structure. The breaking strength of the twine and the nylon line can be increased for use with larger, stronger species.

Having determined that string was a particularly attractive stimulus subsequent experiments were designed to identify those features that were especially influential. Collectively, the results of a series of comparisons demonstrated that chickens were more strongly attracted to stationary bunches of plain white string rather than coloured strings, or ones that incorporated small silver beads (Table 8.1.1). Encouragingly too, despite some waning of interest, bunches of string were still being pecked 17 weeks after their placement in pens containing small groups of one-day-old chicks. Interest in chains and beads had ceased entirely after 6 or 7 days. Furthermore, white string elicited substantial and long-lasting interest by groups of caged laying hens. In this context, it might be worthwhile to consider developing an automated management system that was capable of detecting waning of interest in enrichment devices and then raising them briefly or moving them to a nearby location in an attempt to rekindle interest.

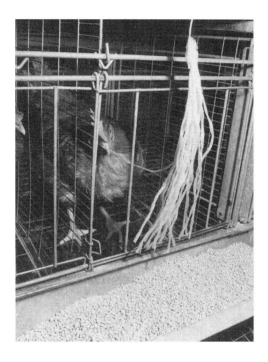

Figure 8.1.1 A string enrichment device readily elicits pecking by laying hens.

Table 8.1.1 Results of systematic comparisons of selected attributes of string enrichment devices

White or yellow	>	green, red, orange or blue
Monochromatic	>	colour combinations
Plain string	>	string with silver beads
Static	>	occasional movement
Size (range: 4x4–16x8 cm)	=	all equally effective

> = elicited greater interest than

A further series of experiments then assessed the effectiveness of the string devices in reducing feather pecking and feather damage. The results are presented concisely in Table 8.1.2 and more fully elsewhere (Blokhuis, Jones, De Jong, Keeling and Preisinger 2001; Jones 2002; Jones, McAdie, McCorquodale and Keeling 2002; Jones, Blokhuis, De Jong, Keeling and Preisinger 2004). Briefly, bunches of string were pecked much more often than hens bearing manipulations of their feathers (e.g., trimming, ruffling) that have been shown to elicit feather pecking (McAdie and Keeling 2000). The provision of string markedly reduced the expression of both gentle and severe feather pecking in an experimental breed known to show very high levels of feather pecking, and it significantly decreased the amount of pecking-related feather damage scored at 30 weeks-of-age in caged groups of laying hens at a commercial farm. The latter effect was apparent regardless of whether the birds had first experienced string when they were just 1 day-old or when they were transferred from rearing to laying cages at 16 weeks-of-age.

Table 8.1.2   Effects of providing string on feather pecking.

- String was pecked more than hens with trimmed / damaged feathers
- String reduced gentle and severe feather pecking in an experimental breed showing high levels of feather pecking
- String reduced pecking-related feather damage in caged layers at a commercial farm

---

Conclusions

The importance of building an enrichment strategy around the birds' preferences cannot be over-emphasised. No claims are made that the provision of string enrichment devices will eradicate the propensity to feather peck and thereby eliminate the need for beak-trimming. However, this form of enrichment is likely to sustain the birds' interest, to promote desirable 'natural behaviours' like exploration and foraging, to potentially reduce boredom, and to significantly reduce the expression of feather pecking as well as the amount of pecking-related feather damage. Each of these effects will contribute to improvements in the birds' welfare, productivity and product quality as well as in public perception of farming practices. String has the added advantages of low cost, durability and ready availability. Its beneficial effects are considered unlikely to be constrained by genotype or housing system because they have already been observed in four different breeds (brown and white), in birds housed singly or in groups and in both cages and floor pens. Encouragingly, string enrichment devices are now being used routinely at a number of commercial farms in Britain and continental Europe.

8.2

Genetics

Joergen B. Kjaer

Introduction

Major changes in poultry production systems have occurred during the last few decades. Genotypes specialised in a very high egg output have been developed (Flock and Heil 2002) and changes in housing and management have been introduced. This has been associated with behavioural problems such as feather pecking and cannibalism, and beak-trimming is used to overcome them. Alternatives to beak-trimming have been sought and genetic selection might be such an alternative. This section will examine the feasibility of this proposal by reviewing papers that have investigated the genetic background of feather pecking and cannibalism. There are many ways of defining these traits, or alternatively, there might be several traits covered under the same term of feather pecking and cannibalism. Therefore a set of such definitions will be the first subject to deal with.

Defining the traits

In general, one can differentiate between self-pecking and allo-pecking. These have been discussed in Chapter 1 but it is worth re-emphasising. If a bird pecks itself, it will normally be preening the feathers, but if the plumage, toes or skin is damaged it is referred to as self pecking or self mutilation. Preening other birds (allo-preening) is pecking the plumage of other birds without doing harm, and is often done in a non-aggressive social context (Harrison 1965) especially in young chicks. Pecking harmfully at other birds is referred to as allo-pecking. Aggressive pecking is forceful allo-pecking usually directed at the facial region (Kruijt 1964). Feathers can be damaged, but it is generally acknowledged that aggressive pecking is not a major cause of feather loss.

Feather pecking ranges in severity from gentle pecking not causing harm to the plumage, to severe feather pecking causing damage or even feather pulling (removal). Feather pulling can result in severe damage of the integument including bleeding from feather follicles (Hughes and Duncan 1972). Distinguishing between severe (damaging) and gentle (non-damaging) pecking can in certain cases be very subjective, and objective methods of classification are still needed.

Birds may be wounded by allo-pecking and even pecked to death. This is called cannibalism and is regarded by some authors as the final phase of severe feather pecking (Bessei 1983; Blokhuis and Arkes 1984; Savory and Mann 1997).

Biometrical studies

Examples of strains and crosses of poultry differing in feather pecking behaviour and mortality due to cannibalism are numerous. From a poultry breeders point of view it is the nature of the genetic components of feather pecking and cannibalism that are interesting and these have not received much attention until recently. Experiments designed for the estimation of genetic parameters have to be extensive. This is due to the properties of variance components, which are the basis of estimating genetic parameters such as heritability. In order to obtain estimates with a reasonable precision, the number of animals has to be large and systematically distributed among sires (males) and dams (females). Individual pedigrees have to be available and observations carried out on individuals or groups of closely related birds. Furthermore, an estimate of heritability is specific for the population on which it is estimated. Therefore estimates can vary quite a bit from one study to the other.

Plumage condition is easy to score on a large number of birds but it is not a precise way of estimating birds tendency to perform feather pecking. Estimates of the heritability of plumage condition range from moderate (0.22) to high (0.54). Direct observation of pecking behaviour is a more precise method of assessing the tendency to perform feather pecking in individuals and has been used in a few experiments to estimate heritability of feather pecking. These estimates range from 0.00 to 0.38. The tendency to receive feather pecking can be measured and heritability estimates for this trait do not differ from zero (Kjaer and Sorensen 1997; Rodenburg, Buitenhuis, Ask, Uitdehaag, Koene, Van der Poel and Bovenhuis 2003). Estimates of heritability for plumage condition and performing feather pecking are shown in Table 8.2.1.

Table 8.2.1 Estimates of heritability of plumage condition and performing feather pecking (FP).

Heritability	SE	Trait	Age (weeks)	Type of exp. (generations of selection)	Reference	Comment
0.54	0.20	Plumage condition	42	Single generation	Damme and Pirchner, 1984	Sire-model
0.23	0.13	Plumage condition	42	Single generation	Damme and Pirchner, 1984	Sire-model
0.37	0.10	Plumage condition	55	Single generation	Craig and Muir, 1989	Sire+dam-model
0.34	0.16	Plumage condition	59	Single generation	Damme and Pirchner, 1984	Sire-model
0.29	0.15	Plumage condition	59	Single generation	Damme and Pirchner, 1984	Sire-model
0.37	0.15	Plumage condition	60	Single generation	Grashorn and Flock 1987	Sire-model
0.22	0.12	Plumage condition	60	Single generation	Grashorn and Flock, 1987	Sire-model
0.22	0.13	Plumage condition	67	Single generation	Damme and Pirchner, 1984	Sire-model
0.30	0.15	Plumage condition	67	Single generation	Damme and Pirchner, 1984	Sire-model
0.06	0.07	No of pecks	6	Single generation	Kjaer and Sorensen, 1997	Sire-model, all FP
0.13	0.07	No of bouts	6	Single generation	Kjaer and Sorensen, 1997	Sire-model, all FP
0.12	0.07	No of gentle bouts	6	Single generation	Rodenburg *et al.* 2003	Animal model
0.00	0.02	No of severe bouts	6	Single generation	Rodenburg *et al.* 2003	Animal model
0.09	0.09	No of pecks	10	Single generation	Cuthbertson, 1980	Heterogeneity chi-square m.
0.07	0.09	No of pecks	18	Single generation	Bessei, 1984	Sire+dam-model
0.15	0.08	No of gentle bouts	30	Single generation	Rodenburg *et al.* 2003	Animal model
0.06	0.05	No of severe bouts	30	Single generation	Rodenburg *et al.* 2003	Animal model
0.14	0.07	No of pecks	38	Single generation	Kjaer and Sorensen, 1997	Sire-model, all FP
0.13	0.07	No of bouts	38	Single generation	Kjaer and Sorensen, 1997	Sire-model, all FP
0.33	0.12	No of pecks	69	Single generation	Kjaer and Sorensen 1997	Sire-model, all FP
0.38	0.12	No of bouts	69	Single generation	Kjaer and Sorensen, 1997	Sire-model, all FP

Table 8.2.1 Contd.

Heritability	SE	Trait	Age (weeks)	Type of exp. (generations of selection)	Reference	Comment
0.20	[1]	No of bouts	28-38	Selection (3)	Kjaer et al. 2001	On combined data from low and high FP-lines
0.18	0.08	No of bouts	28-38	Selection (5)	Su et al. 2003	Low FP-line
0.14	0.07	No of bouts	28-38	Selection (5)	Su et al. 2003)	High FP-line
0.65	0.13	Days without beak-inflicted injury	16-40	Selection (2)	Craig and Muir, 1993	FP, cannibalism and aggression in a combined trait

[1]Realised heritability, no SE given

Selection experiments

Group selection has been very effective in reducing the incidence of beak-inflicted injuries in caged hens (Craig and Muir 1993). The indirect selection criterion was 'hen days without beak-inflicted injuries' which could be regarded as a combined selection against cannibalism, aggression and feather pecking. Divergent selection on individual rate of performing severe feather pecking for two generations on a base population of a commercial laying hybrid produced high and low feather pecking lines significantly different in level of severe feather pecking in generation 1, but in generation 2 there was no significant difference between lines in any type of pecking (gentle or severe feather pecking and aggressive pecking), (Keeling and Wilhelmson 1997).

At the Danish Institute of Agricultural Sciences in Foulum, high and low feather pecking lines have been developed on the basis of a random bred White Leghorn strain maintained as a control line (C). The selection criterion was based on the number of bouts of feather pecking (with no distinction between gentle or severe pecks) recorded during a 3 h observation session in which hens were kept in littered floor pens in groups of 20 consisting of 10 birds from the high pecking line and 10 from the low pecking line. Breeding values were calculated using an Animal Model procedure. After three (Kjaer, Sorensen and Su 2001) and four (Su, Kjaer and Sorensen 2003) generations of selection significant differences in feather pecking behaviour and plumage condition were found between the low and the high pecking line (Figure 8.2.1). Estimates of heritability are given in Table 8.2.1.

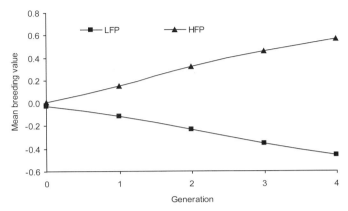

Figure 8.2.1 Mean breeding values of bouts of feather pecking in 4 generations of selected White Leghorn laying hens (Box-Cox transformation scale with l=-0.2). After Su *et al.* (2004)

Indirect selection for and against feather pecking was made at the University of Hohenheim, Germany. Strains of laying hens were selected for or against, pecking at a bunch of feathers connected to an automated recording system (Figure 8.2.2), the 'peck-o-meter' (Bessei, Reiter, Bley and Zeep 1999). The preliminary estimates of heritability in generation 1, 2 and 3 respectively were 0.18, 0.22 and 0.26 (W. Bessei, K. Reiter and A. Harlander-Matauschek, pers. com.). With regard to feather pecking (on live animals) the line selected for a high level of pecking at the feathers of the 'peck-o-meter' showed less feather pecking compared to the line selected for a low level of pecking. This negative phenotypic correlation, estimated to be about –0.30, between pecking at the 'peck-o-meter' and feather pecking is the opposite of the expected relationship according to correlations obtained by (Bessei *et al.*, 1999) and needs further investigation. Other studies have also reported lack of correlation between feather pecking and other behaviour patterns that might have been used for indirect selection (Albentosa, Kjaer and Nicol 2003; P. Hocking, pers. com.) so at the moment only direct selection can be recommended.

Correlated responses to production traits

Genetic correlations are essential in relation to selective breeding in order to understand the effects of selection on one trait, e.g. feather pecking, and the

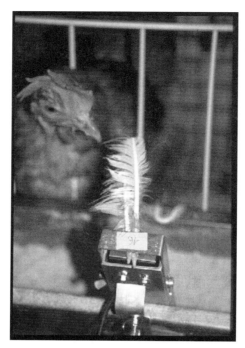

Figure 8.2.2 Automatic recording of pecking to a bunch of feathers, the 'Peck-O-Meter' (Bessei *et al.*, 1999). Photo by J. B. Kjaer.

correlated effect on production and other traits (egg production, sexual maturity etc.). Due to the statistical methods of calculation, genetic correlations mostly have relatively large standard errors and should be treated accordingly. It has been assumed in earlier studies on feather pecking, that selection for high egg production increases the tendency for feather pecking. This relationship is not very clear-cut, however. Selection for and against feather pecking, as described in Kjaer *et al.* (2001) and Su *et al.* (2003), reduced body weight in the low pecking line compared to the high pecking line in generations S3, S5 and S6 (Figure 8.2.3). More precisely the average body weight was reduced in the low pecking line rather than increased in the high pecking line because in generations S4 and S6 the average body weight of the low pecking line was lower than that in the non selected control line, while the average body weight of the high pecking line was not significantly different from that of the control line. Therefore, when selecting against feather pecking, body weight has to be included in the selection index in order to keep the average body weight unchanged. These mechanisms, however, might be different in other lines as estimates are line specific (Falconer 1989). Another difference between the selection lines was found with regard to residual feed consumption. Birds in the low pecking line had better feed efficiency than birds in the high pecking line. This better feed efficiency in the low pecking line is not just due to the lower body weight resulting in a lower requirement for maintenance energy, because residual feed consumption is corrected for differences in body weight. So it is probably due to lower levels of locomotor activity and lower heat loss due to better insulation capacity of the plumage (Su, Kjaer and Sorensen 2004). If this behavioural change is a general one this could mean lower feed to egg costs in lines selected against feather pecking.

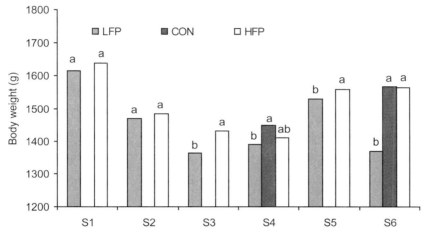

Figure 8.2.3   Body weight as correlated response to selection for HFP and against LFP feather pecking behaviour in White Leghorn. Selection program is described in Kjaer *et al.* (2001). The non-selected control line CON is included in generation S4 and S6. Age at weighing differs between years in the range 28 to 38 weeks. Different letters indicate significant different body weight between lines within generation of selection (S1 to S6). Generation 1 corresponds to generation S1 in Figure 8:2:1 and so forth.

Molecular studies

Biometric studies suggest that the genetic background of feather pecking is polygenic (Kjaer and Sorensen 1997) whereas a major gene may influence the combined trait of cannibalism and aggression (beak-inflicted injuries), (Muir 1996). New molecular techniques have been applied very recently aiming to identify relevant genetic regions or genes that cause differences in feather pecking. Two White Leghorn lines differing in rate of feather pecking, probably due to responses correlated to selection on production parameters (Blokhuis and Beutler 1992) have been the base lines in a two-pronged investigation. A candidate gene and comparative mapping approach address specific genes and supplement the main search for quantitative trait loci (QTL) associated with the target behaviour. In this QTL analysis a screening of 180 microsatellite markers over 600 F_2 birds have been made. Phenotypic recordings on these birds include corticosterone response to manual restraint and observations of feather pecking behaviour in a social test at 6 and 30 weeks-of-age. Suggestive QTL's at genetic loci GGA1 (the chicken chromosome no.1) and GGA2 for gentle (non-damaging) feather pecking at 6 and 30 weeks-of-age have been identified and a significant QTL at GGA2 for severe (damaging) feather pecking was detected at 30 weeks (Buitenhuis, Rodenburg, Van Hierden, Siwek, Cornelissen, Nieuwland, Crooijmans, Groenen, Koene, Korte, Bovenhuis and Van der Poel 2003b). These results suggest that feather pecking behaviour at 6 and 30 weeks may be regulated by different genes and more importantly, that indirect selection to decrease feather pecking and cannibalism by marker-assisted selection may be possible. Also the tendency to receive feather pecking might be genetically regulated. A suggestive QTL was found at GGA2 for receiving gentle feather pecking (Buitenhuis, Rodenburg, Siwek, Cornelissen, Nieuwland, Crooijmans, Groenen, Koene, Korte, Bovenhuis and Van der Poel 2003a). The location on the chromosome was different from the QTL for performing feather pecking which indicates performing and receiving feather pecking are different traits as suggested by Kjaer and Sorensen (1997). These authors did not find any significant heritability for the trait receiving feather pecking in contrast to those of performing feather pecking. Results from a Swedish study (Jensen, Keeling, Schütz, Andersson, Kerje, Carlborg and Jacobsson 2003) supports the hypothesis of separate traits for receiving and performing feather pecking. These authors found no QTL for performing feather pecking in an F_2 population of 751 intercross birds originating from Red Jungle Fowl and White Leghorn. However, a significant QTL was associated with plumage condition reflecting exposure to feather pecking, and this QTL coincided with the colour gene Dominant White. Animals homozygous for the Jungle Fowl allele had significantly poorer plumage condition.

Conclusion

Interest in the genetics of feather pecking and cannibalism has grown in the last few decades and a genetic solution might be more sustainable, efficacious and cost effective than beak-trimming and environmental modifications. Differences in the rate of feather pecking, quality of plumage and mortality from cannibalism between populations of domestic fowl are well documented. The nature of the genetic background of these differences is less well known. Several studies have addressed this question during the past few decades. There is accumulating evidence supporting the existence of additive genetic effects underlying feather pecking behaviour with heritability estimates ranging from 0.0 to 0.4. With regard to cannibalistic pecking there is evidence that one or a few major genes may influence the trait. Selection lines differing in the propensity to perform feather pecking or cannibalistic pecking have been developed. Realised heritabilities of 0.1 to 0.7 have been reported. Correlations between feather pecking behaviour and cannibalistic pecking and traits related to egg production, feed consumption and egg quality need further investigation but are unlikely to be sufficiently high to severely compromise selection for production traits. Correlations to other behavioural traits give reason to believe that indirect selection against feather pecking will not be feasible in the near future. Recent discovery of QTL for performing and receiving feather pecking may offer the opportunity for enhancing the selection intensity. However, the scope is still quite long for these techniques to be commercially attractive and future opportunities to change the propensity for damaging feather pecking and cannibalism in commercial laying hens will meanwhile have to rely on conventional selection in appropriate environments.

Acknowledgements

I want to thank all persons involved in the preparation of earlier versions of this manuscript and in the planning and realisation of the feather pecking selection project at Danish Institute of Agricultural Sciences. Special thanks goes to Werner Bessei, Paul Hocking, Per Isaksen, Bill Muir, Guosheng Su and Poul Sørensen.

8.3

Interaction between nutrition and cannibalism in laying hens

Mingan Choct and Sri Hartini

Introduction

The possibility of preventing cannibalism through dietary manipulation was investigated in the 1940s and 1950s. For example, Bearse, Miller and McClary (1940) and Scott, Holm and Reynolds (1954) found that inclusion of oat hulls in diets decreased the incidence and severity of feather pecking and birds showed superior feather condition. No other studies had been made on the role of nutrition in feather pecking and cannibalism until recently, when several dietary deficiencies were found to be related to feather pecking and/or cannibalism (Cain, Weber, Lockamy and Creger 1984; Cooke 1992; Ambrosen and Petersen 1997). Low levels of dietary protein (Cain *et al.,* 1984; Ambrosen and Petersen 1997), of tryptophan (Shea, Mench and Thomas 1990; Savory, Mann and MacLeod 1999), and of lysine, methionine, and threonine (Ambrosen and Petersen 1997) have been reported to cause aggressive pecking and cannibalism in birds. Diets deficient in phosphorus and sodium have also been linked with the outbreak of cannibalism in chickens (Cooke 1992; Cumming, Chubb, Nolan and Ball 1995). Of particular significance are the findings of Esmail (1997) that addition of oat hulls to a layer diet reduced the incidence of feather pecking and cannibalism in a dose-response manner. Recent research by Hartini, Choct, Hinch, Kocher and Nolan (2002) also found that insoluble dietary fibre was very effective in reducing cannibalism mortality.

Protein and amino acids

Birds consuming diets deficient in protein are often poorly feathered, and an inferior plumage condition can lead to feather pecking and/or cannibalism (Hughes and Duncan 1972; Barnett, Glatz, Newman and Cronin 1997). Cain *et al.* (1984) found that feather pecking in growing pheasants was reduced with dietary protein levels greater than 19%. Ambrosen and Petersen (1997), on the other hand, found no significant effect on the onset of cannibalism or plumage condition in hens with 15.2% or more protein in the diet. It is suggested that an increase in cannibalism when diets low in protein are offered might be due to an imbalance in amino acids, and increasing the protein level would tend to overcome deficiencies in some crucial amino acids. However, when Curtis and Marsh (1993) increased the dietary protein level from 14.5% to 18% by changing the ratio of plant to animal protein feeds, cannibalism mortality increased. They suggested that changes in protein sources might influence the flavour and palatability of the feed, decreasing feed intake and exacerbating the outbreak of cannibalism. March, Biely and Soong (1975) also reported that substituting soybean meal with rapeseed meal as the main protein source for laying hens impaired production efficiency and induced cannibalism. However, recent findings by several workers (Savory *et al.,* 1999; McKeegan, Savory, MacLeod and Mitchell 2001) demonstrated that different dietary protein sources (plant, animal, mainly semi-purified) had no effect on pecking damage in laying hens. This highlights the difficulty in drawing conclusions on whether protein is a predisposing factor for cannibalism because when protein sources are changed, the amount of fibre and anti-nutrients present in the diet will also change.

Fibre

The connection between cannibalism and fibre in poultry comes from the evidence that birds fed oats do not cannibalise each other (Bearse *et al.,* 1940; Scott *et al.,* 1954). This has some support from a study by Wahlstrom, Tauson and Elwinger (1998) who compared the behaviour of birds given a diet based on wheat with that of birds given a diet based on oats. For the wheat and oats diets respectively, total mortalities were 18.4% and 13.4% and deaths from cannibalism were 13.0% and 8.7%.

Oats contain 20-25% non-starch polysaccharides (NSP), with 85-90% being insoluble. The fibre components of poultry diets consist primarily of NSP, which are the main constituents of plant cell walls (Fincher and Stone 1986). In poultry nutrition, however, the focus of research is on the anti-nutritive effect of soluble fibre and little attention has been paid to the roles of insoluble fibre. In an experiment using 1440 non-beak-trimmed ISA Brown laying hens, the effect of diets containing a high level (c. 20%) of insoluble NSP on cannibalism mortality during the pre-lay period (17-20 weeks-of-age) and early-lay period (21-24 weeks-of-age) were investigated. The high fibre diet was more preventative of cannibalism than a commercial diet; mortality was respectively 13.2% vs 3.9% for the pre-lay period and 28.9% vs 14.3% for the early-lay period (Table 8.3.1). When the diets were crossed over, the cannibalism mortality in the flock fed the commercial diet significantly decreased within a week of switching to the high fibre diet. The insoluble fibre source used in this experiment was a wheat by-product (millrun) containing approximately two-thirds bran and one-third pollard. The barley diet was used as a source of soluble fibre as it contains a considerable amount of ß-glucan. Furthermore, an enzyme (ß-glucanase at 300g/kg diet) was used in the barley diet to test if depolymerisation of the polysaccharide would lead to different outcomes for their effect on cannibalism. The confounding factor in this experiment was that the barley diet contained as much insoluble NSP as the millrun diet (11.2% vs. 11.6%). In addition, it also contained 2.1% soluble NSP, which was largely degraded when the enzyme was added to the diet. Thus, the expected difference between the effect of soluble and insoluble fibre on cannibalism was not demonstrated in this study.

Table 8.3.1 Feed intake, egg production and mortality of laying hens fed diets differing in fibre content (Hartini *et al.*, 2002).

| Diets | NSP Level | Mortality (%) | | Early-lay | |
	%	Pre-lay	Early-lay	Feed intake (g/d)	Rate of lay (%)
Wheat	7.2	13.2[b]	28.9[b]	100.6[a]	61.2
Millrun	12.2	3.9[a]	14.3[a]	101.4[a]	64.1
Barley	13.3	5.8[a]	15.9[a]	108.9[b]	63.2
Barley+enzyme	8.9	4.1[a]	17.8[a]	107.8[b]	62.4
P value	<0.01	<0.01	<0.01	<0.01	NS

[ab]Means within a column with different superscripts differ significantly (P<0.05)

Other fibre sources including rice hulls and oat hulls are being tested and are showing a similar effectiveness in controlling cannibalism (Hartini, Choct, Hinch and Nolan 2003). The mechanisms by which high insoluble fibre diets reduce cannibalism in laying hens are not known but a number of hypotheses have been proposed. Firstly, it seems that birds require structural components of feed in the gizzard to regulate downstream digestion of nutrients (Hetland, Choct and Svihus 2004). This is because the modern, highly refined diet that lacks fibre may bypass the crop and the gizzard, leading to a high volume of nutrients, such as starch, entering the small intestine in a short span of time to overwhelm digestive capacity of the bird. This may cause discomfort to the bird which, in turn, could manifest as behavioural changes including cannibalism. Secondly, the transit rate of digesta may play an important role in the outbreak of cannibalism. Since only a limited digestion of insoluble fibre occurs in birds, the side effects will be a more bulky digesta and a shorter residence time of digesta in the gut (Hetland and Choct 2003). The bulking effect of fibre is related to its ability to hold a large amount of water and bacterial mass in its matrix. In our recent study, the rate of feed passage in birds fed wheat, barley and millrun diets was measured using an alkane marker, $C_{36}H_{72}$ (Choct, Hartini, Hinch and Nolan 2002). The maximum excretion of the marker from birds fed the millrun diet occurred during a very short time about 3-4 h after dosing, but occurred during a considerably longer time (3-5 h after dosing) for those fed the wheat diet (Figure 8.3.1). As mentioned earlier, birds fed millrun and barley diets had a lower mortality due to cannibalism than those fed wheat diets (Hartini *et al.*, 2002).

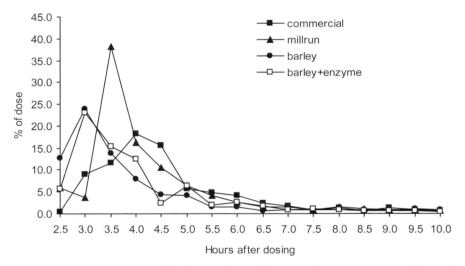

Figure 8.3.1. Alkane excretion per 30-min sampling period expressed as a percentage of the total dose administered during an 8 h complete collection digestion trial (Choct *et al.*, 2002).

It is postulated that a faster rate of digesta passage will stimulate birds to eat more due to the increased need for 'gut fill'. In addition, inclusion of insoluble fibre such as oat hulls reduces energy concentration and birds compensate for this by increasing their feed consumption (Hetland and Svihus 2001). Such a condition may induce birds to spend more time eating and less in pecking each other (Hughes and Black 1977). There is also evidence that birds fed mash diets spend a longer time feeding in order to obtain an adequate amount of energy compared with those fed pellets, and these birds exhibit less pecking behaviour (Aerni, El-Lethey and Wechsler 1999; Aerni, El-Lethey and Wechsler 2000). This seems to support the hypothesis that the bird's drive for energy is an important factor in reducing cannibalism. However, when birds were given a diet containing 4% sand they ate more, and hence spent longer feeding to compensate for the energy dilution, without any reduction in cannibalism mortality (Hartini *et al.,* 2003). It is possible that the bird requires fibre to maintain proper functioning of its gizzard, and hence its 'normal' physiological activities.

Conclusion

An adequate amount of insoluble fibre in the diet appears to be important for minimising the outbreak of cannibalism in chickens. Millrun, oat hulls, rice hulls and lucerne meal are effective sources of fibre in this regard. The mechanisms are probably related to, 1) the physical properties of fibre in modulating the function of the gizzard, giving birds a 'calm feeling', and, 2) increased rate of digesta passage which, in turn, increases the appearance of hunger and results in birds spending more time eating and consequently less time pecking. It is therefore recommended that in order to reduce the occurrence of cannibalism, laying hens should be fed diets containing a high-insoluble fibre, or fed their diet in mash form. A possibility that there is a link between gut microbial status and the outbreak of cannibalism warrants a further study.

8.4

Light intensity

Greg B. Parkinson

Introduction

Manipulation of light intensity, colour and quality in sheds has a direct impact on aggressive pecking and stereotypic behaviours in hens. Low light intensity during the chick rearing stage discourages development of pecking vices.

For many years the clear association between light intensity and cannibalism has been recognised in poultry production (North and Bell 1990; Savory 1995) and higher mortalities through cannibalism are frequently recorded in the top tiers of cages; (North and Bell 1990; Tablante, Vaillancourt, Martin, Shoukri and Estevez 2000) or where light intensities are higher within the shed. More uniform shed light intensities in poultry housing can contribute to lower overall losses through cannibalism (Parkinson 1999; Tablante *et al.,* 2000) and the thresholds for these responses are believed to be between 5-10 lux for conventional incandescent or fluorescent light.

Light colour

The limits of the chicken eye are quite similar to those of humans. All chickens have colour vision and there is some indication that they are able to see better when illumination is by those rays at the long end of the spectrum, such as red, orange and yellow. Colour is the human's perception of different wavelengths of light. Light visible to humans ranges in wavelength from 380 nanometres for violet light to 760 nanometres for red light. A mixture of all the spectral colours produces white light. For humans in bright light, a red and blue object may look equally bright, but under dim light the blue object will appear brighter. In low light vision, the eye is most sensitive to light in the blue hues and is almost blind to red. Thus the advantage of blue light in poultry management is that people can see reasonably well and the birds remain calm (Barnett, Glatz, Almond, Hemsworth, Cransberg, Parkinson and Jongman 2001).

Light quality

The two common types of light are incandescent and fluorescent. Incandescent globes are cheaper to install, have a low light efficiency and have a short life. Compared to incandescent lights, fluorescent lights are 3-4 times as efficient, produce more light for the power used, last about 10 times as long, but have variable performance in cold weather. The colour of the light rays has an effect on the productivity of chickens. For example green and blue light improves growth and lowers age at sexual maturity, while red, orange and yellow light increases age at sexual maturity and red and orange light increase egg production. A part of the difference is thought to be due to the fact that oil droplets in the retina of the eye filter out some of the shorter rays such as green, blue and violet. In spite of these effects, white light is almost entirely used by industry as it represents the best distribution of wavelengths. However, use is made of the fact that birds are calmer in blue light and this is why blue lights are recommended. While birds can distinguish between light sources, for example between low and high frequency fluorescent tubes, there is no evidence that light source impacts on feather pecking and cannibalism (Barnett *et al.,* 2001).

Light intensity

Most commercial egg farms utilise light intensity in the range of 5 to 30 lux in the laying phase, and the effects of the low light intensity in reducing cannibalism, has been attributed primarily to the inability of birds to visualise the cloacal tissue or tissue haemorrhage (Moinard, Morisse and Faure 1990). The other possibility is that the high light intensity may also effect behavioural interactions and trigger aggressive pecking behaviour in birds, irrespective of haemorrhage and injury of birds. Tablante *et al.* (2000) described a 6 fold increase in the incidence of cannibalism between the top and bottom tiers in a two-tier cage system. These differences in mortality were associated with only slight variations in light intensity measured at the feed trough and the authors suggested that cannibalism occurs in clusters with birds in abutting cages adopting these aggressive behaviours.

On commercial egg farms in Australia, 3-fold differences in mortality have been recorded between the top and bottom tiers of cages in 3-4 tier cage systems and are associated with changes in light intensity of between 5 to 35 lux (Parkinson 1999). These differences in mortality have responded to reductions of light intensity in the top tier of cages.

Anecdotal evidence from the egg industry also suggests that pecking and cannibalistic behaviours in pullets is correlated with cannibalistic and pecking behaviours in the laying phase. Effective control of aggressive pecking behaviours in the pullets results in significantly improved control of cannibalism for the flock's life, irrespective of beak-trimming practice.

Recent research at the Primary Industries Research Victoria using 2 flocks (Hatches 1 & 2) of 3 different strains of White Leghorns (A, B, C) has shown a very clear correlation between juvenile pecking and cannibalistic behaviours with subsequent cannibalism in the laying phase (Table 8.4.1).

Table 8.4.1 Mortality and culls due to cannibalism and proportion of flock picked in lines A, B and C between day old and 16 weeks-of-age. Mortality and culls due to cannibalism in lines A, B and C between 16-40 weeks-of-age in two separate hatches housed in the same environment. The light intensity was significantly disrupted at 3 weeks-of-age in Hatch (1) but remained constant in Hatch (2).

Hatch 1 Line	*Mortality (%)*	*Picked (%)*
0-16 weeks		
A	2.5	6.3
B	2.9	5.8
C	0	0
16-40 weeks		
A	5	
B	8	
C	0	

Hatch 2 Line	*Mortality (%)*	*Picked (%)*
0-16 weeks		
A	0	0
B	0	0
C	0	0
16-40 weeks		
A	0	
B	0	
C	0	

Complete control of cannibalism and feather pecking has been achieved in White Leghorn pullets by rearing birds from 1 to 16 weeks-of-age in light intensities of 5 lux using conventional day light entering through fan cowlings (Hatch 2). The precise threshold of light intensity required to achieve this control of pecking and cannibalism is unclear at this stage but believed to be approximately 5-10 lux. The effective control of feather pecking and cannibalism in these young pullets appears to have produced persistent long-term control of cannibalistic behaviours, and supports the experience of many egg producers.

The adoption of controlled environment shedding has significantly reduced the variation in some of the major environmental stressors that have been thought to impact on the induction of cannibalism. These include light intensity, temperature and air quality/humidity. This reduction in environmental variation has significantly improved the ability of the egg industry to achieve control over cannibalism. Several farms have adopted low light intensity housing as a managerial approach to eliminate routine beak-trimming, and have maintained mortality within the normal range despite mild seasonal variation in shed temperature and humidity.

As a more conservative approach, the use of low light intensity rearing has also been combined with more moderate approaches to beak-trimming, such as a first week trim, or a single mild trim to provide producers with additional security against an outbreak of cannibalism.

Experience with flocks that have learnt to feather peck and experienced losses through cannibalism in the growing phase, indicates that it is very difficult to reverse these behaviours even with low light intensity (5 lux) and multiple beak-trimming. Once pecking and cannibalism develops in 2-5 week-old pullets it appears irreversible using current management practices. Beak-trimming and low light intensities are only able to achieve some moderation of the severity of the problem.

The imprinting of feather pecking and cannibalism in pullets may remain a subtle unrecognised feature of some rearing systems that is likely to be responsive to uniformity of light intensity, stocking densities and perhaps some elements of competition, if food and or water access is limiting. Given that feather pecking and cannibalistic behaviours can be completely eliminated from birds in experimental circumstances, the challenge remains to identify the trigger factors that are responsible for the induction of these negative cannibalistic behaviours in many commercial environments.

Additional research on imprinting and management on pecking behaviours may provide new approaches to improve the control of pecking and cannibalism and some insights into techniques in which negative cannibalism behaviours can be reversed

Conclusion

The use of light intensities to modify behaviour provides a powerful tool to improve control of cannibalism, but may not yet be sufficient to justify the complete elimination of beak-trimming as a husbandry practice. In the future, a combination of genetic resistance to these behaviours, combined with imprinting of positive behaviours in production systems that produce consistent control of environmental stress may enable the poultry industry to move away from routine beak-trimming.

8.5

Management of body weight

Greg B. Parkinson

Introduction

Cloacal trauma is one of the most common and severe forms of cannibalism, (Riddell 1991). Most cannibalism occurs between onset of lay and just after peak production (Craig and Lee 1990; Blokhuis and Beuvig 1993). Important predisposing factors have been young poorly developed pullets just coming into lay, obesity and hysteria. Riddell (1991) has suggested that vent pecking is triggered by prolapse or tearing of the vaginal mucosa during passage of an abnormally large egg. The exposure of the cloacal membranes after the expulsion of the egg sometimes attracts other hens to peck at the vent (Appleby, Hughes and Elson 1992). Savory (1995) has also suggested that vent pecking is initiated by a minor prolapse of the uterus immediately after oviposition, exposing the mucous membrane. On the other hand Smith (1982) has suggested that at least 80% of all prolapses result from cannibalistic vent pecking.

Cannibalism also appears to be a learnt behaviour with visual contact between birds triggering clusters of cannibalistic behaviour in caged birds (Appleby *et al.,* 1992; Tablante, Vaillancourt, Martin, Shoukri and Estevez 2000). Whilst other authors have suggested that visualisation of injured birds is an important trigger for cannibalism (Moinard, Morisse and Faure 1990) and is likely to be responsive to light intensity.

Partitioning the effects of tissue damage during egg expulsion from spontaneous aggressive cannibalism may be part of the challenge to improving the capacity of the poultry industry to control cannibalism.

Cloacal haemorrhage

Recent research at the Primary Industries Research Victoria has attempted to define the susceptibility of modern Brown-Egg Layers to cloacal membrane damage during oviposition. Studies using single-bird cages indicates that approximately 10% of normal birds produce blood stained egg shells with some birds exhibiting cloacal haemorrhage. Individual birds are able to rapidly repair the cloacal tissue whereas other birds can produce multiple blood stained eggs with more chronic tissue haemorrhage. Most of the tissue haemorrhage occurs in early egg production and there was a tendency for the problem to be more prevalent in lighter birds producing bigger eggs.

In a controlled study using both normal Heavy (H) and under weight Light (L) pullets, clear evidence was obtained that illustrated the markedly increased susceptibility of under weight birds to early cloacal haemorrhage (Table 8.5.1 and 8.5.2). A 15% reduction in body weight at point of lay was associated with a 3 fold increase in the incidence of cloacal haemorrhage and in the under weight birds about 10% of birds had severe chronic cloacal damage.

Table 8.5.1 Average bodyweight at 36 weeks-of-age of two groups of Brown Egg Layers, normal Heavy (H) and Light (L) housed in single bird cages.

Group	N	Body weight (kg)
L	21	1.65[a]
H	24	2.02[b]

*Means in the same column without a common superscript are significantly different, p<0.05.

Table 8.5.2 Number of birds (36 weeks-of-age) producing blood stained eggs and proportion of blood stained eggs for both bodyweight groups (normal (H) and light (L)).

Group	N	Number of birds laying blood stained eggs	Proportion of blood stained eggs (%)
L	21	9[a]	1.23
H	24	3[b]	0.24

* Means in the same column without a common superscript are significantly different, p<0.05.

Conclusion

Clearly the management of body weight and flock weight distributions can have a profound influence on the incidence of mucosal tearing and cloacal haemorrhage, and could be an important variable in the initiation of cannibalistic behaviours in multiple bird cages.

It has also been hypothesised that vent picking may be the initiating lesion that triggers the onset of salpingitis in the oviduct and perhaps egg peritonitis. Long term studies indicate that salpingitis/egg peritonitis has not been recognised in birds housed in single bird cages, but is common in multiple bird cages (Cumming 2001). Cloacal haemorrhage and vent picking may therefore have consequences for mortality other than the obvious losses through cannibalism.

8.6

Abrasive devices to blunt the beak tip

Thea G.C.M. Fiks-van Niekerk and Arnold Elson

Introduction

Although beak-trimming is performed to minimise feather and injurious pecking in laying hens and thus will reduce stress induced by these behaviours, the treatment itself is a stressor to the birds as well, especially because part of the living tissue of the beak is removed (refer to Chapter 3 and 4). It is however very difficult to mechanically shorten the tip of the beak without touching sensitive beak tissue. Also, the treatment may need to be repeated frequently as the tip can be expected to regrow. In both the Netherlands and the UK research has been conducted to blunt the tip of the beak by using abrasive materials in the feed trough. The idea for beak blunting by abrasion came from claw shortening by abrasion (Tauson 1986; Elson 1990), which has been a requirement of the EU Council Directive 1999/74/EC for laying hens in cages since 01/01/03. A variety of abrasive materials have been found to be effective for claw shortening when fitted to the anti-egg eating baffle plates of laying cages (Niekerk and Reuvekamp 2000; Fiks-van Niekerk, Reuvekamp and Emous 2002; Elson 2003). The idea was that hens blunt the tips of their beaks themselves and will continue to keep the beaks blunt. The reason for placing the abrasive device in the feeder is because hens spend a lot of time pecking the feed, the feed trough and flicking their beaks over the inner surfaces of the feeder.

Dutch pilot trial

In the Netherlands research on beak blunting started with a pilot trial in 1998. Several strips of abrasive material (grain size 60) were attached in the feed trough of a laying cage system (hopper feeder system). The strips had linen underlining and were glued in several positions in the feed trough; onto the vertical side (cage side), onto the bottom, and onto the sloping vertical side (aisle side). These three cages were compared with a cage with no abrasive material. At the end of the laying period the beaks of hens with abrasive material in the feeder were about 1-2 mm shorter (measured from the tip of the beak to the visible line indicating the transition between living tissue and horny tip). The treatment with the abrasive strip fitted to the bottom of the feeder gave the best results. Despite the blunt beaks no difference in feather quality was observed. As the pilot trial was considered promising, a larger trial was set up to investigate effects on mortality and feather cover.

Dutch Large trial

The larger trial was conducted with 1872 non beak-trimmed LSL-hens in 4 different rooms. The hens were all housed on the middle tier of a 3-tier laying cage system (5 hens/cage). Two different light intensities were used; 2 rooms had 14 Lux (=low) and 2 rooms had 38 Lux (=high), measured on the feed trough. All abrasive strips were glued onto the bottom of the feeder, as the pilot trial indicated this as the most successful position.

With the high and low light intensity and the presence or absence of an abrasive strip, there were 4 treatments in total.

Table 8.6.1 shows that the light intensity or the abrasive strip did not influence the production results. There was however an effect on mortality. The highest mortality was observed in the group with the high light intensity and no abrasive strip (HIGH-NO group). Due to the high variation in mortality the statistical analysis only indicated a tendency for a significant difference (P<0.1) between treatments. The lowest mortality was observed in the low light intensity group (with and without abrasive strip; LOW-NO and LOW-STRIP groups) while the group with high light intensity and abrasive strip (HIGH-STRIP) was intermediate.

The abrasive strip did not affect the production responses of birds in the low light intensity group.

Mortality caused by feather pecking and cannibalism showed more pronounced differences. The HIGH-NO group had the highest mortality caused by pecking behaviour (78% of total mortality in this group). In the other groups mortality caused by pecking behaviour was lower (60% of total mortality).

Beak treatment and feather quality

Light intensity did not have any effect on feather quality (Figure 8.6.1). The

Table 8.6.1 Technical results at different light intensities and presence or absence of abrasive strip (18-74 weeks-of-age).

Light intensity	LOW		HIGH	
Abrasive strip	*No*	*Yes*	*No*	*Yes*
% of lay	88.2	88.5	88.0	88.4
Egg weight (g)	61.3	61.0	61.1	61.0
Egg mass (g/h/d)	54.1	54.0	53.7	54.0
Feed intake (g/h/d)	113.8	112.1	113.4	112.3
Kg feed/kg egg	2.11	2.07	2.11	2.08
No. eggs p.h.h.	330.1	332.9	310.4	329.9
Kg eggs p.h.h.	20.25 (a)	20.32 (a)	18.95 (b)	20.13 (a)
Total mortality (%)	9.5 (a)	10.1 (a)	20.7 (b)	13.3 (ab)
Mortality by pecking (%)	5.8 a	6.2 a	16.2 b	7.1 a

Significant differences (P<0.05) are indicated with different letters. Letters in brackets indicate a tendency for a difference (P<0.10). p.h.h. = per hen housed

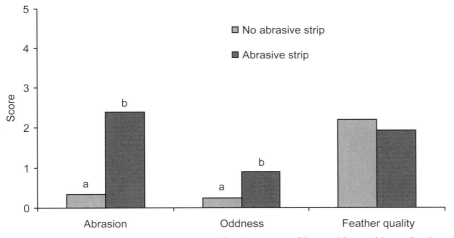

Figure 8.6.1 Abrasion, oddness of beak tips and feather scores of hens with or without abrasive strip in the feed trough (average of scores at 40, 60 and 73 weeks-of-age).

beak tips of the hens with abrasive strips in the feeder were more abraded than beaks of hens without an abrasive strip. The appearance of the blunted beaks was similar to beaks that were trimmed at a very young age. The beaks were not always blunted straight. One side of the beak was often slightly shorter than the other side. It is not likely that hens will feel discomfort because of this, as the oddness was only small (less then 15°) and only occurred on the tip of the beak.

Surprisingly the feather cover was not better for hens with abrasive strips in the feed trough. Apparently the beaks were still long enough to grasp the feathers.

British pilot study

In 2002 the Department for Environment Food and Rural Affairs in the UK set up a beak-trimming action plan to prepare the way for beak-trimming to be phased out by the end of 2010 for pullets in the UK destined for egg production. One aspect of this plan was to carry out a pilot research study assessing alternatives to beak-trimming: beak blunting, at ADAS Gleadthorpe Poultry Research Centre. Work on this project started during 2003 and the current study will be completed in 2005.

From the abrasive materials tested by Elson (2003) in a study on claw shortening, the most effective, and one other, were applied as a coating to most of the inner surface of feed troughs in the Gleadthorpe pilot beak blunting study.

During the rearing period, from 6 to 18 weeks-of-age, four treatments were applied to growing pullets in floor pens. During the laying period, from 18 to 72 weeks-of-age, six treatments are being applied to hens in floor pens and eight treatments to hens in cages. The set-up of the trial is given in table 8.6.2.

Table 8.6.2 Set-up of UK trial.

Treatment in rearing period	Followed by treatment during laying period
1 beak-intact pullets with plain mild steel feed troughs	5 treatment 1 continued
2 beak-intact pullets with troughs coated with abrasive A	6 treatment 2 continued
	7 provision of a plain trough
3 beak-intact pullets with troughs coated with abrasive B	8 treatment 3 continued
	9 provision of a plain trough
4 beak-trimmed pullets (at 8 days old) with plain troughs	10 provision of a trough lined with abrasive C in cages only
	11 provision of a static flat feed chain coated with abrasive B in a plain trough in cages only
	12 treatment 4 continued

Preliminary results

The UK pilot study is ongoing and is being carried out with a single brown hybrid, hence limited information is currently available. A slight degree of beak blunting was evident during rearing and the early part of the laying period in birds on rearing treatments 2 and 3. Birds on rearing treatment 1 generally have the longest beaks followed by those on treatments 2 and 3, which have very slightly shorter ones; those on treatment 4 have considerably shorter and more rounded beaks. These interim results should be viewed with caution until this pilot study has been completed and analysed.

Conclusions

Before drawing any conclusions one should remind readers that only limited results were obtained with one hybrid in the Netherlands and some first impressions of the UK study.

Applying an abrasive strip in the feed trough did blunt the tips of the beaks of laying hens. In the Netherlands this resulted in lower mortality caused by pecking behaviour. The strip did not influence feather cover and production.

The hope in the UK study is that the mild intervention of allowing birds access to abrasives in their feed troughs will remove the sharp tip of the hook of the upper mandible, and that this will result in less damaging feather and flesh pecking. However, whether that aspiration is achieved remains to be seen. If beak blunting does prove to be effective in small-scale studies further research and development will be required:

- to establish whether it is possible to apply the abrasive blunting technique practically and economically on a commercial scale and

- to test its effectiveness in minimising feather pecking and cannibalism in several hybrids in a range of housing systems.

Applying an abrasive strip onto the bottom of the feed trough is not easily possible for chain feeders.

8.7

Use of fitted devices and stock wound sprays

Philip C. Glatz

Introduction

Fitting of light-weight spectacles, use of bitting devices and stock wound sprays were commonly used on birds in the 1960s and 1970s in the poultry industry. Stock wound sprays continue to be used. The rationale for bitting devices was to restrict the vision of the bird and prevent pecking at other birds. Bitting devices are banned in many countries but were utilised extensively in the pheasant industry. Stock wound sprays are commonly used on injuries as a deterrent to prevent birds causing any further damage to the injured bird.

Spectacles

The use of spectacles (anti-pecking devices made of a coloured flexible polyethylene material), when fitted on the nares of the hens allows birds to look to the side or down but not directly ahead. The use of spectacles was effective in controlling feather pecking (Arbi, Cumming and Wodzica-Tomaszewska 1983). Pecking damage was higher for control hens compared to hens with spectacles, which were better feathered after 11 months-of-lay. The use of spectacles has the advantage in reducing social stress by limiting visual contact and breaking down the social hierarchy. Mechanical devices have the same disadvantages. They can only be put on birds of pullet size or larger, they are relatively expensive and they take considerable time to fit to the bird. They cannot be used in cages because they interfere with eating and drinking, can be easily dislodged and these devices are held in place by metal clips which pierce the nasal septum (Robinson 1979).

Contact Lenses

Red contact lenses were first used in the 1960's for layers as an alternative to beak-trimming. They failed to gain popularity because they caused considerable eye irritation, eye infections, abnormal behaviour, and they were not retained well. The lenses were redesigned to eliminate or reduce these problems. The maker of the lenses (Animalens, Inc.) report that lenses have a calming effect on the birds, eliminate the need for beak-trimming, eliminate cannibalism, reduce feed usage and increase egg production. Birds can be fitted with the lenses at the rate of approximately 10 birds/min. Adams (1992) studied the effects of red plastic lenses on egg production, feed per dozen eggs and mortality after being inserted at 12 or 16 weeks-of-age. Egg production was lower and mortality higher, attributed to the inability of birds to find the feed.

Bitting devices

Plastic anti-pecking devices have been developed for use in game birds (Faure, Mellen and Mantovani 1993; Kjaer 1997). They are held in place by lugs inserted in the nares. Studies by Savory and Hetherington (1997) concluded these devices are not commercially applicable to laying hens. In pheasants rings are fitted in the nostril and between mandibles to prevent complete closure of the mandibles. A bumper device protrudes beyond the beak tip to prevent complete closure of the mandibles. The use of bits as a preventative measure against feather pecking is not permitted in many countries (Kjaer 1997).

Tin Pants

Gleaves (1999) reports on the use of 'tin pants' on the vent to minimise vent pecking. The device covered the vent area and prevented other birds from causing injury.

Use of anti-pick compounds

Applying anti-pick compounds (commercial anti-pick, pine tar or axle grease) to wounded areas reduces pecking (Gleaves 1999). In addition application of Vicks vapour rub to wounds prevents further pecking (Grigor, Hughes and Gentle 1995). Studies by Bishop (2001) have also shown that commercially available spays can be applied to wounds and bare areas on the body to improve feather cover.

Vent trauma is probably the biggest cause of mortality in the egg industry. Bishop and Dhaliwal (1994) found mortality from vent pecking and various complications due to vent pecking to be the main cause of death. Parkinson (1990) indicated that vent trauma accounts for between 25 and 50% of the total adult mortality.

Practical experience has shown that treating the everted vent of hens suffering vent trauma with a stock wound spray can rehabilitate these hens. A number of commercial sprays have been tried. Occasionally some of the sprays will leave a stain on the egg.

The practice involves looking for blood stained eggs on the rollout trays each day. Where a blood stained egg is found there is invariably a bird with a traumatised vent. The vent can be readily everted and when the injury is found, it is treated with the stock wound spray. The time to identify a blood stained egg, inspect the hens and spray the vent is about 2 min (Bishop 2001).

Bishop (2001) found that hens beak-trimmed once, had reduced mortality when their vents were sprayed with a stock wound spray. There was no additional benefit when the hens were beak-trimmed twice. Hence stock wound spray is useful for treating vent trauma and may reduce the need for re-trimming. Birds treated with the stock wound spray had better feed conversion and improved egg output as a result of higher egg production and egg weight.

Conclusion

Mechanical devices have disadvantages since they can only be put on birds of pullet size or larger, they are relatively expensive and they take considerable time to fit to the bird.

Lenses, however, have a calming effect on the birds, eliminate the need for beak-trimming, eliminate cannibalism, reduce feed usage and increase egg production.

Plastic anti-pecking devices have been developed for use in game birds but can cause injuries and are banned in many countries.

Practical experience has shown that treating the everted vent of hens suffering vent trauma with a stock wound spray can rehabilitate hens. Mortality can be reduced, and injured hens brought back into production and the need to beak-trim a second time in some strains may be eliminated.

References

Abrahamsson, P., Tauson, R. and Elwinger, K. (1996). Effects on production, health and egg quality of varying proportions of wheat and barley in diets for two hybrids of laying hens kept in different housing systems. *Acta Agricultutae Scandinavica Animal Science* 46: 173-182

Abu-Saad, H. H., Bours, G. J. J. W., Stevens, B. and Hamers, J. P. H. (1998). Assessment of pain in the neonate. *Seminars in Perinatology* 22: 204-416

Adams, R. L. (1992). Effect of red plastic lenses on egg production, feed per dozen eggs, and mortality of laying hens. *Journal of Applied Poultry Research* 1: 212-220

Aerni, V., El-Lethey, L. H. and Wechsler, B. (1999). Feather pecking by laying hens: effects of foraging material and food form. *Aktuelle Arbeiten zur artgemassen Tierhaltung: Vortrage anlasslich der* 30 382: 63-69

Aerni, V., El-Lethey, H. and Wechsler, B. (2000). Effect of foraging material and food form on feather pecking in laying hens. *British Poultry Science* 41: 16-21

Aigner, L. and Caroni, P. (1993). Depletion of 43-kD growth-associated protein in primary sensory neurons leads to diminished formation and spreading of growth cones. *Journal of Cell Biology* 123: 417-429

Akester, A. R. (1979). The autonomic nervous system. In: Form and Function in Birds. King, A. S. and McLelland, J., Academic Press, New York, pp. 388-399

Albentosa, M., Kjaer, J. B. and Nicol, C. J. (2003). Strain and age differences in behaviour, fear response and pecking tendency in laying hens. *British Poultry Science* 44: 333-344

Allen, J. and Perry, G. C. (1975). Feather pecking and cannibalism in a caged layer flock. *British Poultry Science* 16: 441-451

Ambrosen, T. and Petersen, V. E. (1997). The influence of protein level in the diet on cannibalism and quality of plumage of layers. *Poultry Science* 76: 559-563

Anand, K. J. S. and Hickey, P. R. (1987). Pain and its effects in the human neonate and fetus. *New England Journal of Medicine* 317: 1321-1329

Andersen, A. E. and Nafstad, P. H. J. (1968). An electron microscopic investigation of the sensory organs in the hard palate region of the hen (*Gallus domesticus*). *Zeitschrift fur Zellforschung* 91: 391-401

Anderson, K. E. and Davis, G. S. (1997). Performance and fearfulness during the production phase of Leghorn hens reared utilizing alternative beak trimming methods. *Poultry Science* 76: (Suppl. 1): 2 (Abstract)

Andrade, A. N. and Carson, J. R. (1975). The effect of age and methods of debeaking on future performance of White Leghorn pullets. *Poultry Science* 54: 666-674

Angrill, A. and Koster, U. (2000). Psychophysiological stress responses in amputees with and without phantom limb pain. *Physiology and Behaviour* 68: 699-706

Anil, S., Anil, S. L. and Deen, J. (2002). Challenges of pain assessment in domestic animals. *Journal of American Veterinary Medical Association* 220: 313-319

Appleby, M. C. and Hughes, B. O. (1991). Welfare of laying hens in cages and alternative systems; environmental, physical and behavioural aspects. *World's Poultry Science Journal* 47: 109-128

Appleby, M. C., Hughes, B. O. and Elson, H. A. (1992). Poultry Production Systems. Behaviour, Management and Welfare. CAB International, Wellingford

Arbi, A., Cumming, R. B. and Wodzica-Tomaszewska, M. (1983). Effects of vision-restricting polypeepers on the behaviour of laying hens during adaption, feeding, on general activity, agonistic behaviour and pecking damage. *British Poultry Science* 24: 371-381

Arruda, J., Sweitzer, L. S., Rutkowski, M. D. and DeLeo, J. A. (2000). Intrathecal anti-IL-6 antibody and IgG attenuates peripheral nerve injury-induced mechanical allodynia in the rat: possible immune modulation in neuropathic pain. *Brain Research* 879: 216-225

Arulswaminathan, V. S. (1996). Cannibalism in poultry. *Poultry Advisor*: 12-13

Barnett, J. L., Glatz, P. C., Almond, A., Hemsworth, P. H., Cransberg, P. H., Parkinson, G. B. and Jongman, E. C. (2001). Welfare audit for the egg industry. Department of Natural Resources and Environment,Victoria, Australia,

Barnett, J. L., Glatz, P. C., Newman, E. and Cronin, G. M. (1997). Effects of modifying layer cages with solid sides on stress physiology, plumage, pecking and bone strength of hens. *Australian Journal of Experimental Agriculture* 37: 11-18

Barnett, J. L. and Hemsworth, P. H. (2003). Science and its implication in assessing the welfare of laying hens. *Australian Veterinary Journal* 81: 615-623

Barnett, J. L. and Hutson, G. D. (1987). Objective assessment of welfare in the pig: contributions from physiology and behaviour. In: Manipulating Pig Production, Ed. APSA Committee. Australian Pig Science Association: Werribee, Victoria, pp. 1-22

Baron, R. (2000). Peripheral neuropathic pain: from mechanisms to symptoms. *Clinical Journal of Pain* 16 (2 suppl): S12-20

Basbaum, A. I., Julius, D. J. and Robbins, W. R. (2003). Vanilloids. In: Pain

Current Understanding, Emerging Therapies and Novel Approaches to Drug Discovery. Bountra, C., Munglani, R. and Schmidt, W. K., Marcel Dekker Inc., New York, Basel, pp. 531-538

Bateson, P. (1991). Assessment of pain in animals. *Animal Behaviour* 42: 827-839

Bauermann, J. F. (1959). An investigation of the effect of debeaking on feed wastage and fertility of Single Comb White Leghorns. *Poultry Science* 38: 1189 (abstract)

Baum, S. (1995). Characterization and origin of the feather pecking behavioural abnormality. *KTBL Schrift* 370: 97-106

Baxter, M. R. (1994). The welfare problems of laying hens in battery cages. *The Veterinary Record* 134: 614-619

Beane, W. L., Siegel, P. B. and Dawson, J. S. (1967). Size of debeak guide and cauterization time on the performance of Leghorn chickens. *Poultry Science* 46: 1232 (abstract)

Bear, M. F., Connors, B. W. and Paradiso, M. A. (2001). Neuroscience exploring the brain. 2nd ed., Lippincott Williams and Wilkins.

Bearse, G. E., Miller, V. L. and McClary, C. F. (1940). The cannibalism preventing properties of the fibre fraction of oat hulls. *Poultry Science* 18: 210-214

Bell, D. (1996). Can egg producers afford to not beak-trim their flocks? Fourty Fifth Western Poultry Disease Conference, Cancun, Mexico

Bell, D. and Kuney, D. R. (1991). Effect of beak trimming age and high fiber grower diets on layer performance. *Poultry Science* 70: 1105-1112

Bell, D. D. and Adams, C. J. (1998). Environmental enrichment devices for caged layer hens. *Journal of Applied Poultry Research* 7: 19-26

Bennett, G. J. (1993). An animal model of neuropathic pain: a review. *Muscle and Nerve* 16: 1040-1048

Benowitz, L. I. and Routtenburg, A. (1997). GAP-43: an intrinsic determinant of neuronal development and plasticity. *Trends Neuroscience* 20: 84-91

Berkhoudt, H. (1976). The epidermal structure of the bill tip organ in chicks. *Netherlands Journal of Zoology* 26: 561-566

Berkhoudt, H. (1980). The morphology and distribution of cutaneous mechanoreceptors (Herbst and grandry corpuscles) in bill and tongue of the mallard (*Anas platyrhnchos L.*). *Netherlands Journal of Zoology* 30: 1-34

Berryman, J.C. (1986). Parental behaviour in rodents. In: Parental Behaviour (Ed. Sluckin, W. and Herbert, M.), Basil Blackwell Ltd, Oxford, pp. 44-84

Bessei, W. (1983). Zum Problem des Federpickens und Kannibalismus. *Deutsche Geflügelwirtschaft und Schweinproduktion* 24: 656-665

Bessei, W. (1984). Untersuchungen zur Heritabilität des Federpickverhaltens bei Junghennen. 1. Mitteilung. *Archiv fur Geflugelkunde* 48: 224-231

Bessei, W., Reiter, K., Bley, T. and Zeep, F. (1999). Measuring pecking of a bunch of feathers in individually housed hens: first results of genetic studies and feeding related reactions. *Lohmann Information* 22: 27-31

Bilcik, B. and Keeling, L. (1999). Changes in feather condition in relation to feather pecking and aggressive behaviour in laying hens. *British Poultry Science* 40: 444-451

Bishop, R. J. (2001). Controlling vent trauma with stock wound sprays. Publication no 01/090. A report for the Rural Industries Research and Development Corporation

Bishop, R. J. and Dhaliwal, S. (1994). Cage density effects on production and welfare of layers. Proceedings of the 1994 Poultry Information Exchange, Queensland, Australia, pp. 97-106

Blokhuis, H. J. (1986). Feather-pecking in poultry: its relation with ground-pecking. *Applied Animal Behaviour Science* 16: 63-67

Blokhuis, H. J. and Arkes, J. G. (1984). Some observations on the development of feather pecking in poultry. *Applied Animal Behaviour Science* 12: 145-157

Blokhuis, H. J. and Beutler, A. (1992). Feather pecking damage and tonic immobility response in two lines of White Leghorn hens. *Journal of Animal Science* 70: 170

Blokhuis, H. J. and Beuvig, G. (1993). Feather pecking and other characteristics in two lines of laying hens. Proceedings of the Fourth European Symposium on Poultry Welfare, Edinburgh, Scotland, pp. 266-267

Blokhuis, H. J., Jones, R. B., De Jong, I. C., Keeling, L. J. and Preisinger, R. (2001). Feather pecking: solutions through understanding. Report of Seminars. ID-Lelystad, The Netherlands, 37

Blokhuis, H. J. and Metz, J. H. M. (1996). An evaluation on aviary housing for laying hens. Proceedings of the Fifteenth World's Poultry Congress, New Delhi 2: pp. 821-830

Blokhuis, H. J. and van der Haar, J. W. (1989). Effects of floor type during rearing and of beak trimming on ground pecking and feather pecking in laying hens. *Applied Animal Behaviour Science* 22: 359-369

Blokhuis, H. J., van der Haar, J. W. and Koole, P. G. (1987). Effects of beak trimming and floor type on feed consumption and body weight of pullets during rearing. *Poultry Science* 66: 623-625

Blokhuis, H. J. and Wiepkema, P. R. (1998). Studies of feather pecking in poultry. *The Veterinary Quarterly* 20: 6-9

Bloomquist, T. (2001). Amputation and phantom limb pain: a pain-prevention model. *Journal of the American Association of Nurse Anesthetists* 69: 211-217

Bock, R. R. and Samberg, Y. (1990). Vaccination of day-old-chicks against Fowl Pox with the Robot AG-4500. *Israel Journal of Veterinary Medicine* 45(3): 187

Bolton, T. B. (1976). Nervous system. In: Avian Physiology. Sturkie, P. D., Springer-Verlag, New York pp. 1-28

Bourke, M., Glatz, P. C., Barnett, J. L. and Critchley, K. L. (2002). Beak Trimming Training Manual. Edition 1. Publication No. 02/092, Rural Industries Research and Development Corporation

Brambell, F. W. R. (1965). Report of the technical committee to enquire into the welfare of animals kept under intensive livestock husbandry systems. Command Paper No. 28365. HMSO, London

Bray, D. J., Ridlen, S. F. and Gesell, J. A. (1960). Performance of pullets debeaked at various times during the laying year. *Poultry Science* 39: 1546-1550

Breward, J. (1984). Cutaneous nociceptors in the chicken beak. *Journal of Physiology*. London, 346: 56P

Breward, J. (1985). An electrophysiological investigation of the effects of beak trimming in the domestic fowl (*Gallus gallus domesticus*). Ph.D. Thesis, University of Edinburgh

Breward, J. and Gentle, M. J. (1985). Neuroma formation and abnormal afferent nerve discharges after partial beak amputation (beak-trimming) in poultry. *Experientia* 41: 1132-1135

Broom, D. M. and Johnson, K. G. (1993). Stress and strain, welfare and suffering. In: Stress and Welfare. Broom, D. M., Chapman and Hall, London, pp. 143-144

Browder, E. J. and Gallagher, J. P. (1948). Dorsal cordotomy for painful phantom limb. *Annual Surgery* 128: 456-469

Bubien-Waluszewska, A. (1981). The cranial nerves. In: Forms and Function in Birds. Volume 2. King, A. S. and McLelland, J., Academic Press, London, pp. 385-438

Buitenhuis, A. J., Rodenburg, T. B., Siwek, M., Cornelissen, S. J. B., Nieuwland, M. G. B., Crooijmans, R. P. M., Groenen, M. A. M., Koene, P., Korte, S. M., Bovenhuis, H. and Van der Poel, J. J. (2003a). Identification of quantative trait loci for receiving pecks in young and adult laying hens. *Poultry Science* 82: 1661-1667

Buitenhuis, A. J., Rodenburg, T. B., Van Hierden, Y. M., Siwek, M., Cornelissen, S. J. B., Nieuwland, M. G. B., Crooijmans, R. P. M., Groenen, M. A. M., Koene, P., Korte, S. M., Bovenhuis, H. and Van der Poel, J. J. (2003b). Mapping quantative trait loci affecting feather pecking behaviour and stress responses in laying hens. *Poultry Science* 82: 1215-1222

Burchiel, K. J. and Ochoa, J. L. (1991). Pathophysiology of injured axons.

Neurosurgery Clinical North America 2: 105-116

Busnel, M. C. and Molin, D. (1978). Preliminary results of the effects of noise on gestating mice and their pups. In: Effects of Noise on Wildlife. Fletch, J. L. and Busnel, R. G., Academic Press, New York, pp. 209-248

Cabot, P. J. (2001). Immune-derived opioids and peripheral antinociception. *Clinical and Experimental Pharmacology and Physiology* 28: 230-232

Cain, J. R., Weber, J. M., Lockamy, T. A. and Creger, C. R. (1984). Grower diets and bird density effects on growth and cannibalism in ring-necked pheasants. *Poultry Science* 63: 450-457

Campbell, J. N., Raja, S. N., Meyer, R. A. and Mankinnon, S. E. (1988). Myelinated afferents signal the hyperalgesia associated with nerve injury. *Pain* 321: 89-94

Carey, J. B. (1990). Influence of age at final beak trimming on pullet and layer performance. *Poultry Science* 69: 1461-1466

Carey, J. B. and Lassiter, B. W. (1995). Influences of age at final beak trim on the productive performance of commercial layers. *Poultry Science* 74: 615-619

Carson, J. R. (1975). The effect of delayed placement and day-old debeaking on the performance of White Leghorn hens. *Poultry Science* 54: 1581-1584

Carstens, E. (1995). Neuralmechanisms of hyperalgesia: Peripheral and central sensitization? *News Physiology Research* 10: 260-265

Carstens, E. and Moberg, G. P. (2000). Recognizing pain and distress in laboratory animals. *Institute for Laboratory Animal Research* 41: 62-71

Cervero, F. and Laird, J. M. A. (2003). From acute to chronic pain. Peripheral and central mechanisms. In: Current Understanding, Emerging Therapies, and Novel Approaches to Drug Discovery. Bountra, C., Munglani, R. and Schmidt, W., Marcel Dekker Inc., New York, Basel, pp. 29-44

Chen, R., Cohen, L. G. and Hallett, M. (2002). Nervous system reorganization following injury. *Neuroscience* 111: 761-773

Choct, M., Hartini, K., Hinch, G. and Nolan, J. V. (2002). Dietry prevention of cannibalism in layers. *Australian Poultry Science Symposium*, 14: p.157

Chouchkov, C., Palov, A. and Dandov, A. (2002). Ultrastructural immunocytochemistry of calcium-binding proteins in rapidly-adapting avian mechanoreceptors. *Acta Histochemica* 104: 311-320

Coderre, T. J., Katz, J., Vaccarino, A. L. and Melzack, R. (1993). Contribution of central neuroplasticity to pathological pain: a review of clinical and experimental evidence. *Pain* 52: 259-285

Colburn, R. W. and Munglani, R. (2003). Central and peripheral components of neuropathic pain. In: Pain. Current Understanding, Emerging Therapies, and Novel Approaches to Drug Discovery. Bountra, C., Munglani, R. and Schmidt, W., Marcel Dekker Inc., New York, Basel, pp. 45-70

Colburn, R. W., Rickman, A. J. and DeLeo, J. A. (1999). The effect of site and type of nerve injury on spinal glial activation and neuropathic pain behaviour. *Experimental Neurology* 157: 289-304

Cooke, B. C. (1992). Cannibalism in laying hens. *The Veterinary Record* 131: 495

Cooper, J. B. and Barnett, B. D. (1967). Effect of growing regimen and cannibalism control measures on performance of White Leghorn pullets. *Poultry Science* 46: 1443-1447

Craig, J. V. (1992). Beak trimming benefits vary among egg-strain pullets of different genetic stocks. *Poultry Science* 71: 2007-2013

Craig, J. V., Craig, J. A. and Milliken, G. A. (1992). Beak trimming effects on beak length and feed usage for growth and egg production. *Poultry Science* 71: 1830-1841

Craig, J. V. and Lee, H. Y. (1990). Beak-trimming and genetic stocks effects on behaviour and mortality from cannibalism in White Leghorn-type pullets. *Applied Animal Behaviour Science* 25: 107-123

Craig, J. V. and Lee, H.Y. (1989). Research note: Genetic stocks of White Leghorn type differ in relative productivity when beaks are intact versus trimmed. *Poultry Science* 68: 1720-1723

Craig, J. V. and Muir, W. M. (1989). Fearful and associated responses of caged White Leghorn hens: Genetic parameter estimates. *Poultry Science* 68: 1040-1046

Craig, J. V. and Muir, W. M. (1991) Research note: Genetic adaptation to multiple-bird cage environment is less evident with effective beak trimming. *Poultry Science* 70: 2214-2217

Craig, J. V. and Muir, W. M. (1993). Selection for reduction of beak-inflicted injuries among caged hens. *Poultry Science* 72: 411-420

Craig, J. V., Winkler, W. S. M. and Milliken, G. A. (1992). Research Note: Effects of beak trimming and genetic stock on rate of mash consumption and feeding related behaviour in egg-strain pullets. *Poultry Science* 71: 391-394

Cumming, R. B. (2001). The aetiology and importance of salpingitis in laying hens. Proceedings of the Australian Poultry Science Symposium,14: pp.194-196

Cumming, R. B., Chubb, R. C., Nolan, J. V. and Ball, W. (1995). Nutrition and mortality interactions in laying hens. Recent Advances in Animal Nutrition in Australia. Rowe, J. B. and Nolan, J. V., University of New

England, Armidale, Australia, pp. 69-74

Cunha, F. Q. and Ferreira, S. H. (2003). Peripheral hyperalgesic cytokines. *Advances in Experimental Medicine and Biology* 521: 22-39

Cunningham, D. L. (1992). Beak trimming effects on performance, behavior and welfare of chickens: A review. *The Journal of Applied Poultry Research* 1: 129-134

Cunningham, D. L. and Mauldin, J. M. (1996). Cage housing, beak-trimming and induced molting of layers. A review of welfare and production issues. *The Journal of Applied Poultry Research* 5: 63-69

Curtis, P. E. and Marsh, N. W. (1993). Cannibalism in laying hens. *The Veterinary Record* 132: 47-48

Cuthbertson, G. J. (1980). Genetic variation in feather pecking behaviour. *British Poultry Science* 21: 447-450

Damme, K. and Pirchner, F. (1984). Genetic differences of feather-loss in layers and effects on production traits. *Archiv fur Geflugelkunde* 48: 215-222

Deaton, J. W., Lott, B. D., Branton, S. L. and Simmons, J. D. (1987). Research note: Effect of beak trimming on body weight and feed intake of egg-type pullets fed pellets or mash. *Poultry Science* 66: 1552-1554

Del Valle, M. E., Ciriaco, E., Bronzetti, E., Albuerne, M., Naves, F. J., Germana, G. and Vega, J. A. (1995). Calcium-binding proteins in avian Herbst and Grandry sensory corpuscles. *The Anatomical Record* 243: 272-281

Denbow, D. M., Leighton Jr, A. T. and Hulet, R. M. (1984). Behaviour and growth parameters of large white turkeys as affected by floor space and beak trimming. 1. Males. *Poultry Science* 63: 31-37

Desserich, M., Folsch, D. W. and Ziswiler, V. (1984). Das Schnabelkupieren ber Huhnern, Ein Eingriff un innervierten Bereich. *Tierarztliche Praxis* 12: 191-202

Desserich, M., Ziswiler, V. and Folsch, D. W. (1983). Die sensorische Versorgung des Huhnerschnabels. *Revue Suisse Zoology* 90: 799-807

Devor, M. (1994). The pathophysiology of damaged nerves in relation to chronic pain. In: Textbook of Pain. Wall, P. D. and Melzack, R., Churchill Livingstone, Edinburgh, pp. 79-100

Devor, M. (1999). The pathophysiology of damaged nerves in relation to chronic pain. In: Textbook of Pain. Melzack, R., Churchill Livingstone, Edinburgh, pp.79-100

Devor, M. and Rappaport, Z. H. (1990). Pain and the pathophysiology of damaged nerve. In: Pain syndromes in Neurology. Fields, H. L., Butterworths, London, pp. 47-76

Devor, M. and Seltzer, Z. (1999). The pathophysiology of damaged nerves in relation to chronic pain. In: Textbook of Pain (4th ed.), Wall, P. D.

and Melzack, R., Churchill-Livingstone, Edinburgh, pp. 129-164

Dubbeldam, J. L., Bout, R. G. and De Bakker, M. A. G. (1993). An analysis of the trigeminal branches in the beak of normal chickens and after beak trimming, with some behavioural observations. *European Journal of Neuroscience Supplement* 6: 57(abstract).

Dubbeldam, J. L., De Bakker, M. A. G. and Bout, R. G. (1995). The composition of trigeminal nerve branches in normal adult chickens and after debeaking at different ages. *Journal of Anatomy* 186: 619-627

Dubbeldam, J. L. and Den Boer-Visser, A. M. (1993). Immunohistochemical localization of substance P, enkephalin and serotin in the brainstem of chicken, with emphasis on the sensory trigeminal system. *Verhandlungen der Anatomischen Gesellschaft* 88: 7-8

Duncan, I. J. H. and Fraser, D. (1997). Understanding animal welfare. In: Animal Welfare, Appleby, M. C. and Hughes, B. O., CAB International, Oxon, UK, pp. 19-31

Duncan, I. J. H., Slee, G. S., Seawright, E. and Breward, J. (1989). Behavioural consequences of partial beak amputation (beak-trimming) in poultry. *British Poultry Science* 30: 479-488

Eide, P. K. and Rabben, T. (1998). Trigeminal neuropathic pain: pathophysiological mechanisms examined by quantitative assessment of abnormal pain and sensory perception. *Neurosurgery* 43: 1103-1110

Elliot, M. (1995). Factors influencing feathering in commercial pullets and layers. *Poultry Advisor* 28 (5): 45-48

Elson, H. A. (1990). Recent developments in laying cages designed to improve bird welfare. *World's Poultry Science Journal* 46 (1): 34-37

Elson, H. A. (2003). Positive results from claw shortener monitoring. *Poultry World* 157 (8): 14 and 157 (9): 26

Eskeland, B. (1981). Effects of beak trimming. First European Symposium on Poultry Welfare. Danish Branch World's Poultry Science Association, Vester Farimagsgade 1, DK-1606, Copenhagen, Denmark, pp.193-200

Eskeland, B., Bjornstad, S. and Hvidsten, H. (1977). Effect of population density, group size, housing system and beak trimming on production performance of hens in cage and pen. Meld. Nor. Landbrukshogsk (Scientific Reports of the Agricultural University of Norway) 56 (No. 6): 40 pages

Esmail, H. M. (1997). Fiber nutrition. *Poultry International* July: 31-34

Falconer, D. S. (1989). Introduction to Quantitative Genetics, 2nd ed, Longman, New York.

Faure, J. M., Mellen, J. M. and Mantovani, C. C. (1993). Welfare of guinea fowl or game birds. Proceedings of the Fourth European Symposium on Poultry Welfare, Potters Bar, Universities Federation for Animal

Welfare, pp. 148-157

FAWC. (1997). Report on the Welfare of Laying Hens. MAFF. Crown Copyright, PB, 3221

Fiks-van Niekerk, T. G. C. M. (2001). Organic poultry farming: a small but growing concept. Proceedings of the Sixth European Symposium on Poultry Welfare, Zollikofen, Switzerland, pp. 35-37

Fiks-van Niekerk, T. G. C. M., Reuvekamp, B. F. J. and Emous, R. A. v. (2002). Abrasive devices for laying hens in cages. *Archiv fur Geflugelkunde*, Special Issue: abstracts of Eleventh European Poultry Conference, Verlag Eugen Ulmer and Co., Stuttgart p. 145

Fincher, G. B. and Stone, B. A. (1986). Cell walls and their components in cereal grain technology. In: Advances in Cereal Science and Technology Pomeranz, Y., American Association of Cereal Chemists, St Paul, Minnesota, USA, pp. 207-295

Fitzgerald, M. (1983). Capsaicin and sensory neurones - A Review. *Pain* 15: 109-130

Fitzgerald, M. (1994). Neurobiology of fetal and neonatal pain. In: Textbook of Pain (4th Ed), edited by Wall, P.D. and Melzack, R., Churchill-Livingstone, Edinburgh, pp. 153-163

Flock, D. K. and Heil, G. (2002). A long-term analysis of time trends in the performance profile of white-egg and brown-egg hybrid laying strains based on results of official German random sample tets from 1974/75 to 1997/99. *Archiv fur Geflugelkunde* 66: 1-20

Flor, H. (2002). The modification of cortical reorganization and chronic pain by sensory feedback. *Applied Psychophysiology and Biofeedback* 27: 215-227

Flor, H., Devor, M. and Jensen, T. S. (2003). Phantom limb pain: Causes and cures. Proceedings of the Tenth World Congress on Pain, IASP Press, Seattle, pp. 725-738

Frischenschlager, O. and Pucher, L. (2002). Psychological management of pain. *Disability and Rehabilitation* 24: 416-422

Frisen, J., Risling, M. and Fried, K. (1993). Distribution and axonal relations of macrophages in a neuroma. *Neuroscience* 55: 1003-1013

Gaik, G. C. and Farbman, A. I. (1971a). The chicken trigeminal ganglion: I. Fine structure of the neurons during development. *Journal of Morphology* 141: 43-56

Gaik, G. C. and Farbman, A. I. (1971b). The chicken trigeminal ganglion: II. Fine structure of the neurons during development. *Journal of Morphology* 141: 57-76

Ganchrow, D., Gentle, M. J. and Ganchrow, J. R. (1987). Central distribution and efferent origins of facial nerve branches in the chicken. *Brain Research Bulletin* 19: 231-238

Ganchrow, J. and Ganchrow, D. (1986). Chorda tympani innervation of anterior mandibular taste buds in the chicken (*Gallus gallus domesticus*). *Anatomical Record* 216: 434-439

Gao, W., Feddes, J. J. R. and Robinson, F. E. (1994). Effects of stocking density on the incidence of usage of environmental devices by White Leghorn hens. *The Journal of Applied Poultry Research* 3: 336-341

Gargiulo, A. M., Lorvik, S., Ceccarelli, P. and Pedini, V. (1991). Histological and histochemical studies on the chicken lingual glands. *British Poultry Science* 32: 693-702

Gentle, M. J. (1971). The lingual taste buds of *Gallus domesticus L. British Poultry Science* 12: 245-248

Gentle, M. J. (1979). Sensory control of food intake. In: Food Intake Regulation in Poultry. Freedman, B. M., British Poultry Science Ltd., Edinburgh, pp. 259-273

Gentle, M. J. (1983). The chorda tympani nerve and taste in the chicken. *Experientia* 39: 1002-1003

Gentle, M. J. (1984). Sensory functions of the chorda tympani nerve in the chicken. *Experientia* 40: 1253-1255

Gentle, M. J. (1986a). Neuroma formation following partial beak amputation (beak trimming) in the chicken. *Research in Veterinary Science* 41: 383 - 385

Gentle, M. J. (1986b). Beak trimming in poultry. *World's Poultry Science Journal* 42: 268-275

Gentle, M. J. (1989). Cutaneous sensory afferents recorded from the nervus intramandibularis in *Gallus gallus var. domesticus. Journal of Comparative Physiology* A 164: 763-774

Gentle, M. J. (1991). The acute effects of amputation on peripheral trigeminal afferents in *Gallus gallus var. domesticus. Pain* 46: 97-103

Gentle, M. J. (1992). Ankle joint (*Artc. Interarsalis*) receptors in the domestic fowl. *Neuroscience* 49: 991-1000

Gentle, M. J. (1992). Pain in birds. *Animal Welfare* 1: 235-247

Gentle, M. J. (1997). Acute and chronic pain in the chicken. Proceedings of the Fifth European Symposium on Poultry Welfare., Wageningen, Netherlands, pp. 5-12

Gentle, M. J. and Breward, J. (1981). The anatomy of the beak. Proceedings of the First European Symposium on Poultry Welfare, Danish Branch W.P.S.A., pp.185-189

Gentle, M. J. and Breward, J. (1986). The bill tip organ of the chicken (*Gallus gallus var domesticus*). *Journal of Anatomy* 145: 79-85

Gentle, M. J. and Hughes, B. O. (1995). The anatomical and behavioural consequences of beak trimming in turkeys. *Turkeys* April: 23-26

Gentle, M. J., Hughes, B. O., Fox, A. and Waddington, D. (1997). Behavioural and anatomical consequences of two beak trimming methods in 1- and 10-day-old chicks. *British Poultry Science* 38: 453-463

Gentle, M. J., Hughes, B. O. and Hubrecht, R. C. (1982). The effect of beak trimming on food intake, feeding behavior and body weight in adult hens. *Applied Animal Ethology* 8: 147-159

Gentle, M. J. and Hunter, L. N. (1988). Physiological and behavioural responses associated with feather removal in *Gallus gallus var domesticus*. *Research in Veterinary Science* 50: 95-101

Gentle, M. J. and Hunter, L. N. (1993). Neurogenic inflammation in the chicken (*Gallus gallus var domesticus*). *Comparative Biochemistry and Physiology Part C* 105: 459-462

Gentle, M. J., Hunter, L. N. and Waddington, D. (1991). The onset of pain related behaviours following partial beak amputation in the chicken. *Neuroscience Letters* 128: 113-116

Gentle, M. J., Thorp, B. H. and Hughes, B. O. (1995). Anatomical consequences of partial beak amputation (beak trimming) in turkeys. *Research in Veterinary Science* 58: 158-162

Gentle, M. J., Waddington, D., Hunter, L. N. and Jones, R. B. (1990). Behavioural evidence for persistent pain following partial beak amputation in chickens. *Applied Animal Behaviour Science* 27: 149-158

Gibson, S. W., Dun, P. and Hughes, B. O. (1988). The performance and behaviour of laying fowls in a covered strawyard system. *Research and Development in Agriculture* 5: 153-163

Gilmer-Hill, H. S., Beuerman, R., Ma, Q., Jiang, J., Tiel, R. L. and Kline, D. C. (2002). Response of GAP-43 and p75 in human neuromas over time after traumatic injury. *Neurosurgery* 51: 1229-1237

Glatz, P. C. (1987). Effects of beak trimming and restraint on heart rate, food intake, body weight and egg production in hens. *British Poultry Science* 28: 601-611

Glatz, P. C. (1990). Effect of age of beak-trimming on the production performance of hens. *Australian Journal of Experimental Agriculture* 30: 349-355

Glatz, P. C. (2000). Beak trimming methods - a review. *Asian - Australian Journal of Animal Science* 13: 1619-1637

Glatz, P. C. (2004). Laser beak trimming. Final Report to the Australian Egg Corporation Limited.

Glatz, P. C. and Lunam, C. A. (1990). When is the best age to beak trim chickens? Proceedings of the Eighth Australian Poultry and Feed Convention, Gold Coast, Qld. pp. 83-88

Glatz, P. C. and Lunam, C. A. (1994). Production and heart rate responses of chickens beak-trimmed at hatch or at 10 or 42 days-of-age. *Australian*

Journal of Experimental Agriculture 34: 443-447

Glatz, P. C., Lunam, C. A., Barnett, J. L. and Jongman, E. C. (1998). Prevent chronic pain developing in layers subject to beak-trimming and re-trimming. A report to Rural Industries Research and Development Corporation

Glatz, P. C., Murphy, L. B. and Preston, A. P. (1990). Analgesic therapy of beak-trimmed chickens. *Australian Veterinary Journal* 69: 18

Gleaves, J. W. (1999). Cannibalism. Cause and prevention in poultry. WWW article published by Cooperative Extension Institute of Agriculture and Natural Resources, University of Nebraska, Lincoln

Gottschaldt, K. M. (1985). Structure and function of avian somatosensory receptors. In: Form and Function in Birds. Vol 3. King, A. S. and McLelland, J., Academic Press, London, pp. 375-461

Gottschaldt, K. M. and Lausmann, S. (1974). The peripheral morphological basis of tactile sensibility in the beak of geese. *Cell Tissue Research* 153: 477

Grashorn and Flock, D. (1987). Genetisch-Statistische Untersuchungen des Befiederungszustandes an weißen, LSL. und braunen, LB. Hennen. Lohmann Information Nov/Dez: 13-19

Green, L. E., Lewis, K., Kimpton, A. J. and Nicol, C., J. (2000). A cross sectional survey of the prevalence of feather pecking in laying hens and its association with management and disease. *Veterinary Record* 147: 233-238

Greenspan, J. D. (1997). Nociceptors and the peripheral nervous system's role in pain. *Journal of Hand Therapy* 10: 78-85

Gregory, N. G. (1998a). Animal Welfare and Meat Science. CABI Publishing, Oxford, UK, p. 298

Gregory, N. G. (1998b). Decision-making on ethical issues. Vetscript 11 (May), 21.

Grigor, P. N., Hughes, B. O. and Gentle, M. J. (1995). Should turkeys be trimmed? An analysis of the costs and benefits of different methods. *Veterinary Record* 136: 257-265

Guy, J. (2001). Environmental enrichment for broilers - will it prevent feather pecking? *World Poultry* 17 (3): 22-23

Gvaryahu, G. E., Ararat, E., Asaf, E., Lev, M., Weller, J. I., Robinson, B. and Snapir, N. (1994). An enrichment object that reduces aggressiveness and mortality in caged laying hens. *Journal of Physiology and Behaviour* 55(2): 313-316

Hargreaves, R. C. and Champion, L. R. (1965). Debeaking of caged layers. *Poultry Science* 44: 1223-1227

Harrison, C. J. (1965). Allopreening as agonistic behaviour. *Behaviour* 24: 161-209

Hartini, S., Choct, M., Hinch, G., Kocher, A. and Nolan, J. V. (2002). Effects of light intensity during rearing and beak trimming and dietary fiber sources on mortality, egg production, and performance of ISA brown laying hens. *The Journal of Applied Poultry Research* 11: 104-110

Hartini, S., Choct, M., Hinch, G. H. and Nolan, J. V. (2003). Effect of diet composition, gut microbial status and fibre forms on cannibalism in layers. Research Report. The Rural Industries Research and Development Corporation, Canberra, Australia

Hausberger, M. (1992a). Visual pecking preferences in domestic chicks. Part I. Responses of different breeds of chicks to different sorts of seeds. *Academie des Science* 314: 273-278

Hausberger, M. (1992b). Visual pecking preferences in domestic chicks. Part II. Responses of different breeds of chicks to different sorts of seeds. *Academie des Science* 314: 331-335

Heidweiller, J., van Loon, J. A. and Zweers, G. A. (1992). Flexibility of the drinking mechanism in adult chickens (*Gallus gallus, Aves*). *Zoomorphology* 111: 141-159

Hemsworth, P. H. and Barnett, J. L. (1991). The effects of aversively handling pigs either individually or in groups on their behaviour, growth and corticosteroids. *Applied Animal Behaviour Science* 30: 61-72

Hemsworth, P. H., Barnett, J. L. and Campbell, R. G. (1996). A study of the relative aversiveness of a new daily injection procedure for pigs. *Applied Animal Behaviour Science* 49: 389-401

Hemsworth, P. H., Barnett, J. L. and Hansen, C. (1981). The influence of handling by humans on the behaviour, growth and corticosteroids in the juvenile female pig. *Hormones and Behavior* 15: 396-403

Hemsworth, P. H., Barnett, J. L. and Hansen, C. (1986a). The influence of handling by humans in the behaviour, reproduction and corticosteroids of male and female pigs. *Applied Animal Behaviour Science* 15: 303-314

Hemsworth, P. H. and Coleman, G. J. (1998). Human-livestock interactions. In: The Stockperson and the Productivity and Welfare of Intensively Farmed Animals. CAB International, Oxon, UK

Hester, P. Y. and Shea-Moore, M. (2003). Beak trimming egg-laying strains of chickens. *World's Poultry Science Journal* 59: 458-474

Hetland, H., Choct, M. and Svihus, B. (2004). Role of insoluble non-starch polysaccharides in poultry nutrition. *World's Poultry Science Journal* (in press)

Hetland, H. and Svihus, B. (2001). Effect of oat hulls on performance, gut capacity and feed passage time in broiler chickens. *British Poultry Science* 42: 354-361

Hill, J. A. (1986). Egg production in alternative systems-a review of recent research in the UK. *Research and Development in Agriculture* 3: 13-18

Hirt, H. (2001). The influence of group size on the behaviour and welfare of laying hens. Proceedings of the Sixth European Symposium on Poultry Welfare, Zollikofen, Switzerland, pp. 203-208

Holland, G. R. and Robinson, P. P. (1990). The number and size of axons central and peripheral to inferior alveolar nerve injuries in the cat. *Journal of Anatomy* 73: 129-137

Homma, Y., Brull, S. J. and Zhang, J. M. (2002). A comparison of chronic pain behaviour following local application of tumor necrosis factor alpha to the normal and mechanically compressed lumbar ganglia in the rat. *Pain* 95: 239-246

Horch, K. W. and Lisney, S. J. (1981). Changes in primary afferent depolarization of sensory neurons during peripheral nerve regeneration in the cat. *Journal of Physiology* 313: 287-299

Hu, J. W., Sessle, B. J., Raboisson, P., Dallel, R. and Woda, A. (1992). Stimulation of craniofacial muscle afferents induces prolonged facilitatory effects in trigeminal nociceptive brainstem neurons. *Pain* 48: 53-60

Hughes, B. O. and Black, A. J. (1977). Diurnal patterns of feeding and activity in laying hens in relation to dietary restriction and cage shape. *British Poultry Science* 18: 353-360

Hughes, B. O. and Duncan, I. J. H. (1972). The influence of strain and environmental factors upon feather pecking and cannibalism in fowls. *British Poultry Science* 13: 525-547

Hughes, B. O. and Michie, W. (1982). Plumage loss in medium-bodied hybrid hens: the effect of beak-trimming and cage design. *British Poultry Science* 23: 59-64

Hughes, B. O. and Wood-Gush, D. G. (1977). Agonistic behaviour in domestic hens: the influence of housing method and group size. *Animal Behaviour* 25: 1056-1062

Hutson, P. H., Curzon, G. and Trickleband, M. D. (1984). Anti-nociception induced by brief footshock: characterisation and roles of 5-hydroxytryptamine and dopamine. In: Stress Induced Analgesia. Tricklebank, M. D. and Curzon, G., John Wiley and Sons, Chichester, pp. 135-164

Ide, C. and Munger, B. L. (1978). A cytologic study of grandry corpuscle development in chicken toe skin. *Journal of Comparative Neurology* 179: 301-324

Iggo, A. (1984). Pain in Animals. The Hume Memorial Lecture. Universities Federation for Animal Welfare, Wheathampstead, UK

Interagency Research Animal Committee (1985). US government principles for utilization and care of vertebrate animals used in testing, research and training. In: Guide for the Care and Use of Laboratory Animals. Curtis, S. E., Washington DC, pp. 81-83

Jacques, S. and Magali, H. (2001). Nociception and pain related procedures in animal husbandry. Proceedings of the Fifty Second Annual Meeting of the European Association for Animal Production

Jendral, M. J. and Robinson, F. E. (2004). Beak-trimming in chickens: historical, economical, physiological and welfare implications, and alternatives for preventing feather pecking and cannibalistic activity. *Avian and Poultry Biology Reviews* 15: 9-23

Jensen, P., Keeling, L., Schütz, K., Andersson, L., Kerje, S., Carlborg, Ö. and Jacobsson, L. (2003). Feather pecking in poultry-phenotypic correlations and QTL-analysis in an F2-intercross between the Red Jungle Fowl and White Leghorn layers. Proceedings of the Thirty Seventh International Congress ISAE, Abano Terme, Italy, June 24-28, p. 68

Jensen, T. S., Krebs, B., Nielsen, J. and Rasmussen, P. (1983). Phantom limb, phantom pain and stump pain in amputees during the first 6 months following limb amputation. *Pain* 17: 243-256

Jensen, T. S., Krebs, B., Nielsen, J. and Rasmussen, P. (1984). Non-painful phantom limb phenomena in amputees: incidence, clinical characteristics and temporal course. *Acta Neurology Scandinavica* 70: 407-414

Jensen, T. S. and Rasmussen, P. (1994). Phantom pain and related phenomena. In: Textbook of Pain. Wall, P. D. and Melzack, R., Edinburgh, pp. 508-521

Jerrett, S. A. and Goodge, W. R. (1973). Evidence for amylase in avian salivary glands. *Journal of Morphology* 139: 27-46

Ji, R. R. and Woolfe, C. J. (2001). Neuronal plasticity and signal transduction in nociceptive neurons: implications for the initiation and maintenance of pathological pain. *Neurobiology of Disease* 8: 1-10

Johnsen, P. F., Vestergaard, K. S. and Norgaard, N. G. (1998). Influence of early rearing conditions on the development of feather pecking and cannibalism in domestic fowl. *Applied Animal Behaviour Science* 60: 25-41

Jones, R. B. (2001). Environmental enrichment for poultry welfare. In: Integrated Management Systems for Livestock. Wathes, C. M., Occasional Publication of the British Society for Animal Science, 28, pp. 125-131

Jones, R. B. (2002). Role of comparative psychology in the development of effective environmental enrichment strategies to improve poultry welfare. *International Journal of Comparative Psychology* 15: 77-106

Jones, R. B., Blokhuis, H. J., De Jong, I. C., Keeling, L. J. and Preisinger, R. (2004). Feather pecking in poultry: the application of science in a search for a practical solution. *Animal Welfare* 13: S215-S219

Jones, R. B., Carmichael, N. L. and Rayner, E. (2000). Pecking preferences and pre-dispositions in domestic chicks: implications for the development of environmental enrichment devices. *Applied Animal Behaviour Science* 69: 291-312

Jones, R. B., McAdie, T. M., McCorquodale, C. C. and Keeling, L. J. (2002). Pecking at other birds and at string enrichment devices by adult laying hens. *British Poultry Science* 43: 337-343

Jones, R. B. and Ruschak, C. (2002). Domestic chicks' responses to PECKABLOCKS and string enrichment devices. Proceedings of the British Society of Animal Science, p. 215

Jordt, S.-E. and Julius, J. G. (2002). Molecular basis for species-specific sensitivity to "hot" chili peppers. *Cell* 108: 421-430

Kare, M. R. and Rogers, J. G. (1976). Sense organs. In: Avian Physiology. Sturkie, P. D., pp. 29-52

Kathle, J. and Kolstad, N. (1996). Non debeaked laying hens in aviaries. I. Production performance in cages and three types of avaries. *Norwegian Journal of Agricultural Sciences* 10: 413-424

Kavaliers, M., Hirst, M. and Teskey, G. C. (1983). A functional role for an opiate system in snail thermal behavior. *Science* 220: 99-101

Keeling, L. and Wilhelmson, M. (1997). Selection based on direct observations of feather pecking behaviour in adult laying hens. Proceedings of the Fifth Symposium on Poultry Welfare, Wageningen, 7-10 June, pp.77-79

Keeling, L. J. (1995). Feather pecking and cannibalism in layers. *Poultry International* 34: 46-50

Keeling, L. J., Hughes, B. O. and Dun, P. (1988). Performance of free range laying hens in a polythene house and their behaviour on range. Farm Building Progress 94: 21-28

Kennard, D. C. (1937). Chicken vices. Bimonthly Bulletin. 184. Ohio Agricultural Experiment Station 22: 33-39

King, A. S. and McLelland, J. (1975). Outlines of avian anatomy. Bailiere Tindall, London

Kjaer, J. B. (1995). Strain differences in feather pecking behaviour and floor laying in hens kept in Aviaries. Proceedings of the Twenty Ninth International Congress of the International Society for Applied Ethology, Exeter, UK, pp. 191-192

Kjaer, J. B. (1997). Effect of light intensity on growth, feed intake and feather pecking behaviour in beak-trimmed and bitted pheasant chickens (*Phasianus colchivus*). *Archiv fur Geflugelkunde* 61(4): 167-171

Kjaer, J. B. (2001). Genetic aspects of feather pecking and cannibalism. Proceedings of the Sixth European Symposium on Poultry Welfare, Zollikofen, Switzerland, pp. 189-197

Kjaer, J. B. and Sorensen, P. (1997). Feather pecking in White Leghorn chickens - a genetic study. *British Poultry Science* 38: 333-341

Kjaer, J. B., Sorensen, P. and Su, G. (2001). Divergent selection of feather pecking behaviour in laying hens (*Gallus gallus domesticus*). *Applied Animal Behaviour Science* 71: 229-239

Kjaer, J. B. and Vestergaard, K. S. (1999). Development of feather pecking in relation to light intensity. *Applied Animal Behaviour Science* 62: 243-254

Klemm, R., Reiter, K. and Pingel, H. (1995). Investigations on feather pecking in muscovy ducks. *Archiv fur Geflugelkunde* 59: 99-102

Kostarczyk, E. (1999). Recent advances in neonatal pain research. *Folia Morphology* 58: 47-56

Kruijt, J. P. (1964). Ontogeny of social behaviour in Burmese red junglefowl (*Gallus Gallus spadiceus*). *Behaviour Supplement* 12: 1-201

Kuney, D. R. and Bell, D. D. (1982). Effects of beak trimming method and cage density on laying hens. Progress in Poultry through Research. University of California Cooperative Extension, May Issue (No. 24.)

Kuo, F.-L., Craig, J. V. and Muir, W. M. (1991). Selection and beak-trimming effects on behavior, cannibalism, and short term production traits in White Leghorn pullets. *Poultry Science* 70: 1057-1068

Lawson, S. N. (1995). Neuropeptides in morphologically and functionally identified primary afferent neurons in dorsal root ganglia: Substance P, CGRP and somatostatin. In: Progress in Brain Research. Volume 104, Nyberg, F., Sharma, H. and Wiesenfeld-Hallin, Z., Elsevier Science, pp. 161-173

Lay, Jr., D. C., Friend, T. H., Grissom, K. K., Bowers, C. L. and Mal, M. E. (1992). Effects of freeze or hot-iron branding of Angus calves on some physiological and behavioural indicators of stress. *Applied Animal Behaviour Science* 33: 440-446

Lee, B. H. (2002). Managing pain in human neonates - applications for animals. *Journal of American Veterinary Medical Association* 221: 233-237

Lee, H. Y. and Craig, J. V. (1990). Beak-trimming effects on the behavior and weight gain of floor-reared, egg strain pullets from three genetic stocks during the rearing period. *Poultry Science* 69: 568-575

Lee, H. Y. and Craig, J. V. (1991). Beak-trimming effects on behavior patterns, fearfulness, feathering, and mortality among three stocks of White Leghorn pullets in cages or floor pens. *Poultry Science* 70: 211-221

Lee, K. (1980). Long term effects of Marek's disease vaccination with cell-free Herpes virus of turkey and age at debeaking on performance and mortality of White Leghorns. *Poultry Science* 59: 2002-2007

Lee, K. and Moss, C. W. (1995). Effects of cage density on fear-related behavioural reponse and activity of layers. *Poultry Science* 74: 1426-1430

Lee, K. and Reid, I. S. (1977). The effects of Marek's disease vaccination and day-old debeaking on the performance of growing pullets and laying hens. *Poultry Science* 56: 736-740

Leighton, Jr., A. T., Denbow, D. M. and Hulet, R. M. (1985). Behaviour and growth parameters of large white turkeys as affected by floor space and beak trimming. II. Females. *Poultry Science* 64: 440-446

Lervik, S., Oppermann Moe, R., Tauson, R., Hetland, H. and Svihus, B. (2001). Preliminary experiences with furnished cages in Norway. Proceedings of the Sixth European Symposium on Poultry Welfare, Zollikofen, Switzerland, pp. 23-25

Ley, S. J., Livingstone, A. and Waterman, A. E. (1989). The effect of chronic clinical pain on thermal and mechanical threshold in sheep. *Pain* 39: 353-357

Ley, S. J., Waterman, A. E. and Livingstone, A. (1995). A field study of the effect of lameness on mechanical nococeptive thresholds in sheep. *Veterinary Record July*, 22: 85-87

Lindenmaier, P. and Kare, M. R. (1959). The taste end-organs of the chicken. *Poultry Science* 38: 545-550

Lu, Y., Park, T., Rice, F. L. and Laurito, C. E. (2003). Absence of substance P and CGRP in the dorsal root ganglia of naked mole rats correlates with an absense of hyperalgesia to heat. Proceedings of the Tenth World Congress on Pain, 24, pp. 227-234

Lucas, A. M. and Stettenheim, P. R. (1972). Avian Anatomy. Integument., U.S.D.A Agriculture Handbook 362, Washington DC.

Lunam, C. A. and Gentle, M. J. (2004). Substance P immunoreactive nerve fibres in the domestic chick ankle joint before and after acute arthritis. *Neuroscience Letters* 354: 87-90

Lunam, C. A. and Glatz, P. C. (1993). Taste buds of the domestic fowl are innervated by nerve fibres immunoreactive for calbindin but not for substance P. Australian Neuroscience Symposium, p.115

Lunam, C. A. and Glatz, P. C. (1995a). Overcoming chronic pain in beak-trimmed poultry. Egg Industry Research and Development Council, UFZE, pp. 54

Lunam, C. A. and Glatz, P. C. (1995b). Substance P and calcitonin gene-related peptide in the upper beak of the chicken with particular reference to the salivary glands. Proceedings of the Australian Poultry Science Symposium, University of Sydney, p.176

Lunam, C. A. and Glatz, P. C. (2000). Declawing of farmed emus-harmful or helpful. Rural Industries Research and Development Corporation, pp. 43

Lunam, C. A., Glatz, P. C. and Barnett, J. L. (1998). Neuroma formation in layers after re-trimming. Proceedings of the Australian Poultry Science Symposium 10: p. 206

Lunam, C. A., Glatz, P. C. and Hsu, Y.-J. (1996). The absence of neuromas in beaks of adult hens after conservative trimming at hatch. *Australian Veterinary Journal* 74: 46-49

Lyon Electric Company Inc. (1982). A general guide to beak-trimming. Bulletin No. 144

Maizama, D. G. and Adams, A. W. (1994). Effect of beak-trimming, blade temperature, and age at beak-trimming on performance of two strains of egg layers. *The Journal of Applied Poultry Science* 3: 69-73

March, B. E., Beily, J. and Soong, R. (1975). The effects of rapeseed meal during the growing and/or laying periods on mortality and egg production in chickens. *Poultry Science* 54: 1875-1882

Mason, J. R. and Maruniak, J. A. (1983). Behavioural and physiological effects of capsaicin in red-winged blackbirds (*Agelaius phoeniceus*). *Pharmacology, Biochemistry and Behaviour* 19: 857-862

McAdie, T. M. and Keeling, L. J. (2000). Effect of manipulating feathers of laying hens on the incidence of feather pecking and cannibalism. *Applied Animal Behaviour Science* 68: 215-229

McBride, G. (1971). Crowding without stress. *Australian Veterinary Journal* 47: 564-567

McFarlane, J. M. and Curtis, S. E. (1989). Multiple concurrent stressors in chicks. 3. Effects on plasma corticosterone and the heterophil: lymphocyte ratio. *Poultry Science* 68: 522-527

McFarlane, J. M., Curtis, S. E., Shanks, R. D. and Carmer, S. G. (1989a). Multiple concurrent stressors in chicks.1. Effect on weight gain, feed intake, and behaviour. *Poultry Science* 68: 501-509

McFarlane, J. M., Curtis, S. E., Simon, J. and Izquierdo, O. A. (1989b). Multiple concurrent stressors in chicks. 2. Effects on hematologic, body composition, and pathologic traits. *Poultry Science* 68: 510-521

McHugh, J. M. and McHugh, W. B. (2000). Pain: neuroanatomy, chemical mediators, and clinical implications. *AACN Clinical Issues* 11: 168-178

McIntosh, J. I., Slinger, S. J., Sibbald, I. R. and Ashton, G. C. (1962). The effects of three physical forms of wheat on the weight gains and feed effeciencies of pullets from hatching to fifteen weeks of age. *Poultry Science* 41: 438-445

McKeegan, D. E. F. and Savory, C. J. (1999). Feather eating in layer pullets and its possible role in the aetiology of feather pecking damage. *Applied Animal Behaviour Science* 65: 73-85

McKeegan, D. E. F., Savory, C. J., MacLeod, M. G. and Mitchell, M. A. (2001). Development of pecking damage in layer pullets in relation to dietary protein source. *British Poultry Science* 42: 33-42

McNeill, T. H., Mori, N. and Cheng, H. W. (1999). Differential regulation of the growth-associated proteins, GAP-43 and SCG-10, in response to unilateral cortical ablation in adult rats. *Neuroscience* 90: 1349-1360

Megret, S., Rudeaux, F., Faure, J. M. and Picard, M. (1996). The role of the beak in poultry. Effects of debeaking. *INRA Production Animals* 9(2): 113-119

Melzack, R. and Wall, P. D. (1965). Pain mechanisms: A new theory. *Science* 150: 971-979

Mench, J. A. (1992). The welfare of poultry in modern production systems. *Poultry Science Reviews* 4: 107-128

Mense, S. (1983). Basic neurobiologic mechanisms of pain and analgesia. *American Journal of Medicine* 75: 4-14

Merskey, H. and Bogduk, N. (1994). Classification of chronic pain. In: Desciptions of Chronic Pain Syndromes and Definitions of Pain Terms (2nd ed.), IASP Press, Seattle

Michie, W. and Wilson, C. W. (1985). The perchery system for housing layers. The Scottish Agricultural Colleges Research and Development Note

Millan, M. J. (1999). The induction of pain: an integrative review. *Progress in Neurobiology* 37: 1-164

Moinard, C., Morisse, J. P. and Faure, J. M. (1990). Effect of cage area, cage height and perches on feather condition, bone breakage, and mortality in laying hens. *British Poultry Science* 59: 198-202

Moiniche, S., Dahl, J. B. and Kehlet, H. (1993). Time course of primary and secondary hyperalgesia after heat injury to the skin. *British Journal of Anaesthia* 71: 201-205

Molony, V. (1992). Is animal pain the same as human pain? In: Animal Pain: Ethical and Scientific Perspectives. Kuchel, T. R., Rose, M. and Burrell, J., Australian Council on the Care of Animals in Research and Teaching, Glen Osmond, SA, Australia

Molony, V. and Kent, J. E. (1997). Assessment of acute pain in farm animals using behavioural and physiological measurements. *Journal of Animal Science* 75: 266-272

Morgan, W. (1957). Effect of day-old debeaking on the performance of pullets. *Poultry Science* 36: 208-210

Mousa, S. A. (2003). Morphological correlates of immune-medicated peripheral opioid analgesia. *Advances in Experimental Medicine and Biology* 521: 77-87

Muir, W. M. (1996). Group selection for adaption to multiple-hen cages: Selection program and direct responses. *Poultry Science* 75: 447-458

Nafstad, P. H. J. (1971). Comparative ultrastructural study on merkel cells and dermal basal cells in poultry (*Gallus domesticus*). *Zeitschrift fur Zellforschung* 116: 342-348

Narsinghani, U. and Anand, K. J. S. (2000). Developmental neurobiology of pain in neonatal rats. *Laboratory Animals* 29: 27-39

Nickel, R., Schummer, A. and Seiferle, E. (1977). Anatomy of the domestic birds., Verlag Paul Parey, Berlin, Hamburg

Nicol, C. J., Lewis, K., Poetzsch, C. and Green, L. E. (2001). A case-control study investigating factors for feather pecking in free-range hens. Proceedings of the Sixth European Symposium on Poultry Welfare, Zollikofen, Switzerland, pp. 244-249

Niekerk, T. G. C. M. v. and Reuvekamp, B. F. J. (2000). Abrasive strips for laying hens: how can we get a durable, effective device? *World Poultry* 16 (4): 16-17

Nixey, C. (1994). Lighting for the production and welfare of turkeys. *World's Poultry Science Journal* 50: 292-294

Noble, D. O. and Kestor, K. E. (1997). Beak-trimming of turkeys. 2. Effects of arc trimming on weight gain, feed intake, feed wastage, and feed conversion. *Poultry Science* 76: 668-670

Noble, D. O., Muir, F. V., Krueger, K. K. and Nestor, K. E. (1994). The effect of beak-trimming on two strains of commercial tom turkeys. 1. Performance traits. *Poultry Science* 73: 1850-1857

Noden, D. M. (1980). Somatotopic and functional organization of the avian trigeminal ganglion: Horseradish peroxidase analysis in the hatching chick. *Journal of Comparative Neurology* 190: 405-428

Nolen, R. S. (2001). The ethics of pain management in animals. *Journal of American Veterinary Medical Association* 219: 1661

Norgaad-Nielsen, J., Kjaer, G. and Simonsen, H. B. (1993). Afprovning af to alternative aegproduktions-systemer-Hans Kier Systemet og Boleg II systemet. Statens Husdyrbrugsforsog Forskningsrapport 9/1993

North, M. O. and Bell, D. B. (1990). Commercial Chicken Production Manual, 4th Edition. Reinhold, V. N., New York

O'Malley, P. (1999). Declawing emu chicks. Final report to Rural Industries Research and Development Corporation.

Parkinson, G. B. (1990). Prolapse and Vent trauma-Still a problem in laying hens? Proceedings of the Eighth Australian Poultry and Feed Convention, Queensland, Australia, pp. 89-95

Paul-Murphy, J. and Ludders, J. W. (2001). Avian analgesia. *Veterinary Clinic of North American Exotic Animal Practice* 4: 35-45

Peckham, M. C. (1984). Vices and miscellaneous diseases and conditions.

In: Diseases of Poultry, Edition 8, Iowa State University Press, Ames, Iowa, USA, pp. 741-782

Pickett, I. J. (1969). Debeaking of poultry. *Journal of Agriculture* 72: 417-419

Pierau, F.-K., Gamse, R., Harti, G. and Gamse, R. (1987). Neuropeptides in sensory neurons of pigeons and the insensitivity of avians to capsaicin. In: Fine Afferent Nerve Fibres and Pain. Schmidt, R. F., Schaible, H.-G. and Vahle-Hinz, C., Verlags-gesellschaft, Weinheim pp. 215-223

Pitcher, G. M. and Henry, J. L. (2000). Cellular mechanisms of hyperalgesia and spontaneous pain in a spinalized rat model of peripheral neuropathy: changes in myelinated afferent inputs implicated. *European Journal of Neuroscience* 12: 2006-2020

Polley, C. R., Craig, J. V. and Bhagwat, A. L. (1974). Crowding and agonistic behaviour: a curvilinear relationship? *Poultry Science* 53: 1721-1723

Puchalski, M. and Nummel, P. (2002). The reality of neonatal pain. *Advances in Neonatal Care* 2: 233-244

Renner, P. A., Nestor, K. E. and Havenstein, G. B. (1989). Effects of turkey mortality and body weight of type of trimming, age at beak-trimming, and injection of poults with vitamin and electrolyte solution at hatching. *Poultry Science* 68: 369-373

Rice, A. S. C. and Casale, R. (1994). Microneurography and the investigation of pain mechanisms. *Pain Reviews* 1: 121-137

Richards, M. P. M. (1966). Maternal behaviour in virgin female golden hamsters (*Mesocricetus auratus* Waterhouse): the role of the age of the test pup. *Animal Behaviour* 14: 303-309

Riddell, C. (1991). Developmental, metabolic and miscellaneous disorders. Iowa State University Press, Ames, IA, p. 827

Robertson, K. E., Cross, P. J. and Terry, J. C. (1985). The crucial first days. *American Journal of Nursing* 85: 30-47

Robinson, D. (1979). Effects of cage shape, colony size, floor area, and cannibalism prevention on laying performance. *British Poultry Science* 20: 345-356

Robinson, L. (1961). Modern Poultry Husbandry. Temperton, H., Crosby Lockwood and Sons Ltd, London

Rodenburg, T. B., Buitenhuis, A. J., Ask, B., Uitdehaag, K. A., Koene, P., Van der Poel, J. J. and Bovenhuis, H. (2003). Heritability of feather pecking and open-field response in laying hens at two different ages. *Poultry Science* 82: 861-867

Saito, I. (1966). Comparative anatomical studies of the oral organs of the poultry. V. Structures and distribution of taste buds of the fowl. *Bulletin of the Faculty of Agriculture University Miyazaki* 13: 95-102

Sandilands, V. and Savory, C. J. (2002). Ontogeny of behaviour in intact and beak trimmed layer pullets, with special reference to preening. *British Poultry Science* 43: 182-189

Sanford, J., Ewbank, R., Molony, V., Tavernor, W. D. and Uvarov, O. (1986). Guidelines for the recognition and assessment of pain in animals. *Veterinary Record* 118: 334-338

Sann, H., Harti, G., Pierau, F.-K. and Simon, E. (1987). Effect of capsaicin upon afferent mechanisms of nociception and temperature regulation in birds. *Canadian Journal of Physiology* 65: 1347-1354

Sann, H. and Pierau, F.-K. (1998). Efferent functions of C-fiber nociceptors. *Zeitschrift fur Rheumatologie* 57: 8-13

Savory, C. J. (1995). Feather pecking and cannibalism. *World's Poultry Science Journal* 51: 215-219

Savory, C. J. and Hetherington, J. D. (1997). Effects of anti-pecking devices on food intake and behaviour of laying hens fed on pellets or mash. *British Poultry Science* 38: 125-131

Savory, C. J. and Mann, J. S. (1997). Behavioural development in groups of pen-housed pullets in relation to genetic strain, age and food form. *British Poultry Science* 38: 38-47

Savory, C. J., Mann, J. S. and MacLeod, M. G. (1999). Incidence of pecking damage in growing bantams in relation to food form, group size, stocking density, dietary trytophan concentration and dietary protein. *British Poultry Science* 40: 579-584

Saxod, R. (1978). Ultrastructure of merkel corpuscles and so-called "transitional" cells in the white leghorn chicken. *American Journal of Anatomy* 151: 453-474

SCARM (1995). Model Code of Practice for the Welfare of Animals. Domestic Poultry. Standing Committee of Agriculture and Resources Management. CSIRO Publications, Victoria, Australia.

Schafer, M. (2003). Cytokines and peripheral analgesia. *Advances in Experimental Medicine and Biology* 521: 40-50

Schafer, M., Carter, L. and Stein, C. (1994). Interleukin 1 beta and corticotropin-releasing factor inhibit pain by releasing opioids from immune cells in inflamed tissue. Proceedings of National Academy of Sciences (U.S.A.) 91: pp. 4219-4223

Schott, G. D. (2001). Delayed onset and resolution of pain: some observations and implications. *Brain* 124: 1067-1076

Schwob, J. E., Youngentob, S. L. and Meiri, K. F. (1994). On the formation of neuromata in the primary olfactory projection. *Journal of Comparative Neurology* 340: 361-380

Scott, M. I., Holm, J. S. and Reynolds, R. E. (1954). Studies on pheasant nutrition. 2. Protein and fiber levels in diets for young pheasants. *Poultry Science* 33: 1237-1244

Seetha Rama Rao, V. (1988). Vices in a commercial broiler farm. *Poultry Advisor*, 21, pp. 29-31

Shea, M. M., Mench, J. A. and Thomas, O. P. (1990). The effect of dietary trytophan on aggressive behaviour in developing and mature broiler breeder males. *Poultry Science* 69: 1664-1669

Sheen, K. and Chung, J. M. (1993). Signs of neuropathic pain depend on signals from injured nerve fibers in a rat model. *Brain Research* 610: 62-68

Shirley, H. V. (1977). The influence of the method of debeaking on the incidence of impacted beaks in chickens. *Tennessee Farm and Home Science Progress Report* 103: 12-13

Slinger, S. J. and Pepper, W. F. (1964). Effects of debeaking and feeding whole grain on the reproductive performance of pullets. *Poultry Science* 43: 356-362

Slinger, S. J., Pepper, W. F. and Sibbald, I. R. (1962). The effects of debeaking at eight weeks of age on the grit consumption, weight gains and feed efficiencies of growing pullets. *Poultry Science* 41: 1614-1615

Smith, J. A. and Boyd, K. M. (1991). Lives in the Balance: the Ethics of using Animals in Biomedical Research. Oxford, Oxford University Press

Smith, R. (1982). Debeaking management can minimise blowout losses. *Feedstuffs*, April, pp.10-11

Smith, T. W. (1997). Miscellaneous management related diseases. Cooperative Extension Service, Mississippi State University

Sneddon, L. and Gentle, M. J. (1992). Pain in farm animals. *Animal Welfare* 1: 235-247

Sommerhoff, G. (1990). Life, Brain and Consciousness. Amsterdam, North Holland

Stasiak, K. L., Maul, D., French, E., Hellyer, P. W. and VandeWoude, S. (2003). Species-specific assessment of pain in laboratory animals. *Contemporary Topics in Laboratory Animal Science* 42: 13-20

Stevens, V. I., Blair, R., Salmon, R. E. and Stevens, J. P. (1984). Effect of varying levels of dietary vitamin D3 on turkey hen egg production, fertility and hatchability, embryo mortality and incidence of embryo beak malformations. *Poultry Science* 63: 760-764

Stokes, W. S. (2000). Reducing unrelieved pain and distress in labotatory animals using humane endpoints. *Institute for Laboratory Animal Research* 4: 59-61

Struwe, F. J., Gleaves, E. W., Douglas, J. H. and Bond, P. L. (1992a). Effect of rearing floor type and ten-day beak trimming on stress and performance of caged layers. *Poultry Science* 71: 70-75

Struwe, F. J., Gleaves, E. W. and Douglas, J. H. (1992b). Stress measurements on beak-trimmed and untrimmed pullets. *Poultry Science* 71: 1154-1162

Su, G., Kjaer, J. B. and Sorensen, P. (2003). Genetic improvement on feather pecking behaviour is effective. Proceedings of the Third European Poultry Genetics Symposium, 17-19 September, Wageningen, Holland, p.84

Su, G., Kjaer, J. B. and Sorensen, P. (2004). Selection for feather pecking behaviour has changed feed efficiency. Proceedings of the Twenty Fifth World's Poultry Congress, June, Istanbul, Turkey

Sundaresan, K. and Jayaprasad, I. A. (1979). The art of debeaking chickens. *Poultry Advisor*, January, pp. 45-47

Sundaresan, K., Jayaprasad, I. A. and Kothandaraman, P. (1979). The effect of debeaking at different stages on the growing performance of White Leghorn pullets. *Cheiron* 8: 149-152

Szolcsanyi, J., Sann, H. and Pierau, F.-K. (1986). Nociception in pigeons is not impaired by capsaicin. *Pain* 27: 247-260

Tablante, N. L., Vaillancourt, J. P., Martin, S. W., Shoukri, M. and Estevez, I. (2000). Spatial distribution of cannibalism mortalities in commercial laying hens. *Poultry Science* 79: 705-708

Tal, M. (1999). A Role for Inflammation in Chronic Pain. *Current Review of Pain 3*: 440-446

Tal, M., Wall, P. D. and Devor, M. (1999). Myelinated afferent fiber types that become spontaneously active and mechanosensitive following transection in the rat. *Brain Research* 824: 218-223

Tanaka, T. and Yoshimoto, T. (1985). Tampering with food by laying hens. *Japanese Journal of Zootechnology Science* 56: 994-996

Tauson, R. (1986). Avoiding excessive growth of claws in caged laying hens. *Acta Agriculturae Scandinavica* 36: 95-106

Tauson, R. and Abrahamsson, P. (1992). Keeping systems for laying hens-effects on production, health, behaviour and working environment. Proceedings of the Nineteeth World's Poultry Congress, Amsterdam (2): pp. 327-332

Tauson, R. and Holm, K.-E. (2001). First furnished small group cages for laying hens in evaluation program on commercial farms in Sweden. Proceedings of the Sixth European Symposium on Poultry Welfare, Zollikofen, Switzerland, pp. 287-288

Treede, R. D. (1995). Peripheral acute pain mechanisms. *Annals of Medicine* 27: 213-216

Underwood, W. J. (2002). Pain and distress in agricultural animals. *Journal of the American Veterinary Medical Association* 221: 208-211

United Egg Producers Animal Husbandry Guidelines for U.S. Egg Laying Flocks (2002). Alpharetta, GA, p. 4

Van Hierden, Y. M., Korte, S. M., Ruesink, E. W., Van Reenen, C. G., Engel, B., Koolhaas, J. and Blokhuis, H. J. (2002a). The development of feather pecking behaviour and targeting of pecking in chicks from a high and low feather pecking line of laying hens. *Applied Animal Behaviour Science* 77: 183-196

Van Hierden, Y. M., Korte, S. M., Ruesink, E. W., Van Reenen, C. G., Engel, B., Korte-Bouws, G. A., Koolhaas, J. M. and Blokhuis, H. J. (2002b). Adrenocortical reactivity and central serotonin and dopamine turnover in young chicks from a high and low feather pecking line of laying hens. *Physiology and Behaviour* 75: 653-659

Van Liere, P. (1995). Responsiveness to a novel preening stimulus long after partial beak amputation (beak trimming) in laying hens. *Behavioural Processes* 34: 169-174

Van Rooijen, J. and Blokhuis, H. J. (1990). The quality of beak-trimming. Proceedings of Summer Meeting Society for Veterinary Ethology, Pistoia, Italy, p. 115

Van Rooijen, J. and Haar, J. W. V. D. (1997). Comparison of laser trimming with traditional beak-trimming at day 1 and week 6. Proceedings of the Fifth European Symposium on Poultry Welfare, Wageningen, The Netherlands, pp. 141-142

Vatine, J. J., Argov, R. and Seltzer, Z. (1998). Brief electrical stimulation of c-fibers in rats produces thermal hyperalgesia lasting weeks. *Neuroscience Letters* 246: 125-128

Vestergaard, K. S. 1994. Dustbathing and its relation to feather pecking in the fowl: motivational and development aspects. Thesis. The Royal Veterinary and Agricultural University, Copenhagen, 150 p

Wahlstrom, A., Tauson, R. and Elwinger, K. (1998). Effects on plumage condition, health and mortality of dietary oats/wheat ratios to three hybrids of laying hens in different housing system. *Acta Agriculture Scandinavica* 48: 250-260

Walker, A. W. and Elson, A. (2001). Furnished laying cages: preliminary findings from a research study at ADAS Gleadthorpe. Proceedings of the Sixth European Symposium on Poultry Welfare, Zollikofen, Switzerland, pp. 17-19

Walker, J. S. (2003). Anti-inflammatory effects of opioids. *Advances in Experimental Medicine and Biology* 521: 148-160

Wall, P. D. (1979). Three phases of evil: the relation of injury to pain. Ciba Foundation Symposium, 69: pp. 293-304

Wall, P. D. (1981). On the origin of pain associated with amputation. Siegfried, J. and Zimmermann, M., Springer Verlag, Berlin, pp. 2-14

Wall, P. D. (1983). Alterations in the central nervous system after deafferentation: connectively control. In: Advances in Pain Research and Therapy. Bionica, J. J., Lindblom, U. and Iggo, A., Raven Press, New York, pp. 677-689

Wall, P. D. (1991). Neuropathic pain and injured nerve: central mechanisms. *British Medical Bulletin* 47: 631-643

Wall, P. D. (1992). Defining pain in animals. In: Animal Pain. Short, C. E. and VanPoznak, A., Churchill Livingstone, New York, USA, pp. 63-79

Wechsler, B., Huber, E. B. and Nsh, D. R. (1998). Feather pecking in growers: A study with individually marked birds. *British Poultry Science* 39: 178-185

Weinstein, S. M. (1998). Phantom limb pain and related disorders. *Neurologic Clinics* 16: 919-936

Wells, R. (1983). Beak-trimming. Is it really necessary? World Poultry, June, pp. 28-31

Wilfred, R., Joseph, S. A. and Jeganathan, G. (1982). A simple inexpensive device for debeaking poultry. *Cheiron* 11: 2

Wood-Gush, D. G. M. (1959). A history of the domestic fowl from antiquity to the 19th century. *Poultry Science* 38: 321-326

Workman, L. and Rogers, L. J. (1990). Pecking preferences in young chickens: effects of nutritive reward and beak trimming. *Applied Animal Behaviour Science* 6: 115-126

Wu, J. and Chiu, D. T. (1999). Painful neuromas: a review of treatment modalities. *Annual Plastic Surgery* 43: 661-667

Yamamoto, T., Nagai, T., Shimura, T. and Yasoshima, Y. (1998). Roles of chemical mediators in the taste system. *Japanese Journal of Pharmacology* 76: 325-348

Yannakopoulos, A. L. and Tserven-Gousi, A. S. (1986). Egg shell quality as influenced by 18-day beak trimming and time of oviposition. *Poultry Science* 65: 398-400

Zayan, R. (1986). Assessment of pain in animals: epistemological comments. In: Assessing Pain in Farm Animals. Duncan, I. J. H. and Molony, V., Office for Official Publications of the European Communities, Luxembourg, pp.1-14

Zimmermann, M. (2001). Pathobiology of neuropathic pain. *European Journal of Pharmacology* 429: 23-37

Index